Tinnitus: Imaging, Endovascular and Surgical Approaches

Editors

PRASHANT RAGHAVAN
DHEERAJ GANDHI

NEUROIMAGING CLINICS
OF NORTH AMERICA

www.neuroimaging.theclinics.com

Consulting Editor
SURESH K. MUKHERJI

May 2016 • Volume 26 • Number 2

ELSEVIER

1600 John F. Kennedy Boulevard • Suite 1800 • Philadelphia, Pennsylvania, 19103-2899

http://www.neuroimaging.theclinics.com

NEUROIMAGING CLINICS OF NORTH AMERICA Volume 26, Number 2
May 2016 ISSN 1052-5149, ISBN 13: 978-0-323-44473-6

Editor: John Vassallo (j.vassallo@elsevier.com)
Developmental Editor: Casey Jackson

Neuroimaging Clinics of North America (ISSN 1052-5149) is published quarterly by Elsevier Inc., 360 Park Avenue South, New York, NY 10010-1710. Months of issue are February, May, August, and November. Business and editorial offices: 1600 John F. Kennedy Blvd., Suite 1800, Philadelphia, PA 19103-2899. Business and editorial offices: 6277 Sea Harbor Drive, Orlando, FL 32887-4800. Periodicals postage paid at New York, NY, and additional mailing offices. Subscription prices are USD 365 per year for US individuals, USD 564 per year for US institutions, USD 100 per year for US students and residents, USD 415 per year for Canadian individuals, USD 718 per year for Canadian institutions, USD 525 per year for international individuals, USD 718 per year for international institutions and USD 260 per year for Canadian and foreign students and residents. To receive student/resident rate, orders must be accompanied by name of affiliated institution, date of term, and the *signature* of program/residency coordinator on institution letterhead. Orders will be billed at individual rate until proof of status is received. Foreign air speed delivery is included in all *Clinics* subscription prices. All prices are subject to change without notice. POSTMASTER: Send address changes to *Neuroimaging Clinics of North America*, Elsevier Health Sciences Division, Subscription **Customer Service, 3251 Riverport Lane, Maryland Heights, MO 63043. Telephone: 1-800-654-2452 (U.S. and Canada); 314-447-8871 (outside U.S. and Canada). Fax: 314-447-8029. E-mail: journalscustomer** service-usa@elsevier.com **(for print support);** journalsonlinesupport-usa@elsevier.com **(for online support).**

Reprints. For copies of 100 or more of articles in this publication, please contact the Commercial Reprints Department, Elsevier Inc., 360 Park Avenue South, New York, NY 10010-1710. Tel.: 212-633-3874; Fax: 212-633-3820; E-mail: reprints@ elsevier.com.

Neuroimaging Clinics of North America is covered by *Excerpta Medical/EMBASE,* the RSNA Index of Imaging Literature, *MEDLINE/PubMed (Index Medicus),* MEDLINE/MEDLARS, SciSearch, Research Alert, and Neuroscience Citation Index.

PROGRAM OBJECTIVE

The goal of *Neuroimaging Clinics of North America* is to keep practicing radiologists and radiology residents up to date with current clinical practice in radiology by providing timely articles reviewing the state of the art in patient care.

TARGET AUDIENCE

Practicing radiologists, radiology residents, and other healthcare professionals who utilize neuroimaging findings to provide patient care.

LEARNING OBJECTIVES

Upon completion of this activity, participants will be able to:
1. Review the neuroscience of tinnitus.
2. Discuss the imaging and diagnosis of tinnitus.
3. Recognize endo-vascular and surgical interventions in the management of tinnitus.

ACCREDITATION

The Elsevier Office of Continuing Medical Education (EOCME) is accredited by the Accreditation Council for Continuing Medical Education (ACCME) to provide continuing medical education for physicians.

The EOCME designates this enduring material for a maximum of 15 *AMA PRA Category 1 Credit*(s)™. Physicians should claim only the credit commensurate with the extent of their participation in the activity.

All other health care professionals requesting continuing education credit for this enduring material will be issued a certificate of participation.

DISCLOSURE OF CONFLICTS OF INTEREST

The EOCME assesses conflict of interest with its instructors, faculty, planners, and other individuals who are in a position to control the content of CME activities. All relevant conflicts of interest that are identified are thoroughly vetted by EOCME for fair balance, scientific objectivity, and patient care recommendations. EOCME is committed to providing its learners with CME activities that promote improvements or quality in healthcare and not a specific proprietary business or a commercial interest.

The planning committee, staff, authors and editors listed below have identified no financial relationships or relationships to products or devices they or their spouse/life partner have with commercial interest related to the content of this CME activity:

Todd Abruzzo, MD; Sameer A. Ansari, MD, PhD; Carol A. Bauer, MD; David J. Eisenman, MD; Girish M. Fatterpekar, MD; Anjali Fortna; Dheeraj Gandhi, MBBS, MD; Joseph J. Gemmete, MD, FACR, FSIR; Ronna Hertzano, MD, PhD; Ferdinand K. Hui, MD; Timothy R. Miller, MD; Suresh K. Mukherji, MD, MBA, FACR; Prashant Raghavan, MBBS; Tanya Rath, MD; Michael A. Reardon, MD; Daniel Ryan, MD; Erin Scheckenbach; Yafell Serulle, MD; Christian L. Stanton, MD; Andrew Steven, MD; Karthik Subramaniam; Taylor B. Teplitzky, BS; John Vassallo; Sean Woolen, MD.

UNAPPROVED/OFF-LABEL USE DISCLOSURE

The EOCME requires CME faculty to disclose to the participants:
1. When products or procedures being discussed are off-label, unlabelled, experimental, and/or investigational (not US Food and Drug Administration [FDA] approved); and
2. Any limitations on the information presented, such as data that are preliminary or that represent ongoing research, interim analyses, and/or unsupported opinions. Faculty may discuss information about pharmaceutical agents that is outside of FDA-approved labelling. This information is intended solely for CME and is not intended to promote off-label use of these medications. If you have any questions, contact the medical affairs department of the manufacturer for the most recent prescribing information.

TO ENROLL

To enroll in the *Neuroimaging Clinics of North America* Continuing Medical Education program, call customer service at 1-800-654-2452 or sign up online at http://www.theclinics.com/home/cme. The CME program is available to subscribers for an additional annual fee of USD 235.

METHOD OF PARTICIPATION

In order to claim credit, participants must complete the following:
1. Complete enrolment as indicated above.
2. Read the activity.
3. Complete the CME Test and Evaluation. Participants must achieve a score of 70% on the test. All CME Tests and Evaluations must be completed online.

CME INQUIRIES/SPECIAL NEEDS

For all CME inquiries or special needs, please contact elsevierCME@elsevier.com.

NEUROIMAGING CLINICS OF NORTH AMERICA

ISSUE OF RELATED INTEREST

Radiologic Clinics of North America, January 2015 (Vol. 53, No. 1)
Head and Neck Imaging
Richard H. Wiggins and Ashok Srinivasan, *Editors*
Available at: http://www.radiologic.theclinics.com

THE CLINICS ARE AVAILABLE ONLINE!
Access your subscription at:
www.theclinics.com

Contributors

CONSULTING EDITOR

SURESH K. MUKHERJI, MD, MBA, FACR
Professor and Chairman, Walter F. Patenge
Endowed Chair, Chief Medical Officer and
Director of Health Care Delivery, Michigan
State University Health Team, Department of
Radiology, Michigan State University, East
Lansing, Michigan

EDITORS

PRASHANT RAGHAVAN, MBBS
Division of Neuroradiology, Department of
Diagnostic Radiology and Nuclear Medicine,
University of Maryland School of Medicine,
Baltimore, Maryland

DHEERAJ GANDHI, MBBS, MD
Professor and Director, Division of
Interventional Neuroradiology; Professor,
Departments of Radiology, Neurology and
Neurosurgery University of Maryland School
of Medicine, Baltimore, Maryland

AUTHORS

TODD ABRUZZO, MD
Department of Neurosurgery, Mayfield Clinic
and Cincinnati Children's Hospital, University
of Cincinnati, Cincinnati, Ohio

SAMEER A. ANSARI, MD, PhD
Departments of Radiology, Neurology and
Neurological Surgery, Northwestern University,
Illinois

CAROL A. BAUER, MD
Professor and Chair, Division of
Otolaryngology, Department of Surgery,
Southern Illinois University School of Medicine,
Springfield, Illinois

DAVID J. EISENMAN, MD
Associate Professor, Department of
Otorhinolaryngology–Head and Neck Surgery,
University of Maryland School of Medicine,
Baltimore, Maryland

GIRISH M. FATTERPEKAR, MD
Associate Professor, Department of Radiology,
NYU Langone Medical Center, New York,
New York

DHEERAJ GANDHI, MBBS, MD
Professor and Director, Division of
Interventional Neuroradiology; Professor,
Departments of Radiology, Neurology and
Neurosurgery University of Maryland School
of Medicine, Baltimore, Maryland

JOSEPH J. GEMMETE, MD, FACR, FSIR
Professor, Departments of Radiology,
Neurosurgery and Otolaryngology, University
of Michigan Health System, Ann Arbor,
Michigan

RONNA HERTZANO, MD, PhD
Assistant Professor, Department of
Otorhinolaryngology–Head and Neck Surgery,
University of Maryland School of Medicine,
Baltimore, Maryland

FERDINAND K. HUI, MD
Department of Radiology, Johns Hopkins University, Baltimore, Maryland

TIMOTHY R. MILLER, MD
Assistant Professor of Radiology, Division of Interventional Neuroradiology, Department of Diagnostic Radiology, University of Maryland School of Medicine, Baltimore, Maryland

PRASHANT RAGHAVAN, MBBS
Division of Neuroradiology, Department of Diagnostic Radiology and Nuclear Medicine, University of Maryland School of Medicine, Baltimore, Maryland

TANYA RATH, MD
Assistant Professor, Department of Radiology, University of Pittsburgh School of Medicine, Pittsburgh, Pennsylvania

MICHAEL A. REARDON, MD
Neuroradiology Division, Department of Radiology and Medical Imaging, University of Virginia, Charlottesville, Virginia

DANIEL RYAN, MD
Resident Physician, Department of Diagnostic Radiology, Memorial Medical Center, Southern Illinois University School of Medicine, Springfield, Illinois

YAFELL SERULLE, MD, PhD
Division of Interventional Neuroradiology, Department of Diagnostic Radiology, University of Maryland School of Medicine, Baltimore, Maryland

CHRISTIAN L. STANTON, MD
Neuroradiology Fellow, Department of Radiology, NYU Langone Medical Center, New York, New York

ANDREW STEVEN, MD
Division of Neuroradiology, Department of Diagnostic Radiology and Nuclear Medicine, University of Maryland School of Medicine, Baltimore, Maryland

TAYLOR B. TEPLITZKY, BS
Department of Otorhinolaryngology–Head and Neck Surgery, University of Maryland School of Medicine, Baltimore, Maryland

SEAN WOOLEN, MD
Department of Radiology, University of Michigan Health System, Ann Arbor, Michigan

Contents

Tinnitus is a consequence of changes in auditory and nonauditory neural networks following damage to the cochlea. Homeostatic compensatory mechanisms occur after hearing loss and these mechanisms alter the balance of excitatory and inhibitory neurotransmitters. In many individuals with hearing loss, chronic tinnitus and related phenomena emerge. Some people with tinnitus are disturbed by this subjective sensation. When auditory network dysfunction is coupled with limbic-gating dysfunction, an otherwise meaningless auditory percept such as tinnitus may acquire negative emotional features. The development of effective treatment options is enhanced by the understanding of the neural networks underpinning tinnitus.

The clinical evaluation of patients with tinnitus differs based on whether the tinnitus is subjective or objective. Subjective tinnitus is usually associated with a hearing loss, and therefore, the clinical evaluation is focused on an otologic and audiologic evaluation with adjunct imaging/tests as necessary. Objective tinnitus is divided into perception of an abnormal somatosound or abnormal perception of a normal somatosound. The distinction between these categories is usually possible based on a history, physical examination, and audiogram, leading to directed imaging to identify the underlying abnormality.

Tinnitus is an auditory perception of internal origin. Tinnitus is not a diagnosis but a symptom with many possible causes and correspondingly divergent pathophysiologic, anatomic, diagnostic, and therapeutic considerations. This article provides a summary of the imaging findings of structural causes of tinnitus.

Tinnitus is a common symptom that usually originates in the middle ear. Vascular causes of pulsatile tinnitus are categorized by the location of the source of the noise within the cerebral-cervical vasculature: arterial, arteriovenous, and venous. Arterial stenosis secondary to atherosclerotic disease or dissection, arterial anatomic variants at the skull base, and vascular skull base tumors are some of the more common causes of arterial and arteriovenous pulsatile tinnitus. Noninvasive imaging is indicated to evaluate for possible causes of pulsatile tinnitus, and should be followed by catheter angiography if there is a strong clinical suspicion for a dural arteriovenous fistula.

Pulsatile tinnitus from intracranial venous abnormalities is an uncommon cause of pulse synchronous tinnitus. Endovascular therapies may have applications in many of these disease conditions. They have the advantage of being minimally invasive and may selectively eliminate the site of turbulence. Venous stenting has been used successfully to treat venous stenoses with low complication rates and high success rates in patients with idiopathic intracranial hypertension though randomized controlled data are lacking. Careful exclusion of other causes of tinnitus should be performed before consideration for surgical or endovascular treatment of presumed causative lesions of venous tinnitus.

Although tinnitus may originate in damage to the peripheral auditory apparatus, its perception and distressing symptomatology are consequences of alterations to auditory, sensory, and limbic neural networks. This has been described in several studies, some using advanced structural MR imaging techniques such as diffusion tensor imaging. An understanding of these complex changes could enable development of targeted treatment. New MR imaging techniques enabling detailed depiction of the labyrinth may be useful when diagnosis of Meniere disease is equivocal. Advances in computed tomography and MR imaging have enabled noninvasive diagnosis of dural arteriovenous fistulae.

Foreword
Tinnitus

 CrossMark

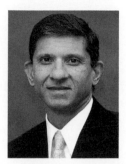

Suresh K. Mukherji, MD, MBA, FACR
Consulting Editor

Tinnitus has been a challenging topic for centuries. When I was "growing up," we classified tinnitus as "subjective" versus "objective," "pulsatile" versus "continuous," or whether there was a retrotympanic mass. The answer to these questions directly affected the imaging evaluation and differential diagnosis. However, the various classifications created much confusion about this topic and led to inconsistent management and treatment of this important disorder.

I sincerely thank Drs Prashant Raghavan and Dheeraj Gandhi for tackling this perplexing subject. This issue delves into the biologic basis of this disease and focuses on the recent advances in neuroscience that have shed new light on the neural basis of this complex disorder. They have taken a unique approach and have focused this issue on the clinical aspects of tinnitus, imaging evaluation, and the various surgical and endovascular techniques used in current and future treatment strategies.

This is really a unique perspective on this disease, and I thank Drs Raghavan and Gandhi for taking this distinct approach. I also thank the article authors for their marvelous contributions.

This is an issue that will "stand the test of time" and be a benchmark reference on this subject for many years.

Finally, I have to personally thank and acknowledge Dr Dheeraj Gandhi. I had the pleasure of having Dheeraj as one of my fellows when I was at University of Michigan. We were fortunate to have him as a faculty member before he was later recruited to Johns Hopkins. Dheeraj is now Professor and Chief of Neurointerventional Radiology at University of Maryland. Dheeraj has been a wonderful colleague and friend over the past 15 years. His rapid rise is a combination of intellect, talent, and most importantly, his humanity. Thank you very much, Dheeraj!

Suresh K. Mukherji, MD, MBA, FACR
Department of Radiology
Michigan State University
Health Care Delivery
Michigan State University Health Team
846 Service Road
East Lansing, MI 48824, USA

E-mail address:
mukherji@rad.msu.edu

http://dx.doi.org/10.1016/j.nic.2016.03.002
1052-5149/16/$ – see front matter © 2016 Published by Elsevier Inc.

neuroimaging.theclinics.com

Preface
Tinnitus—More Than Ringing in the Ears

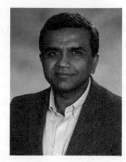 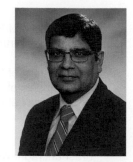

Prashant Raghavan, MBBS   Dheeraj Gandhi, MBBS, MD

Editors

Tinnitus is not merely ringing in the ears. It is a condition that has distressed many a great mind—from the Spanish master, Francisco Goya, to Charles Darwin, to Pete Townshend of The Who, among many, many others. It is an incredibly common ailment, afflicting millions worldwide and is a key symptom in survivors of traumatic brain injury. Tinnitus is the single most common service-related disability reported by veterans. The focus of this issue of the *Neuroimaging Clinics* is on the clinical aspects of tinnitus, its imaging evaluation, and surgical and endovascular techniques used in its treatment. This issue delves also into recent advances in neuroscience that have shed new light on the neural basis of this complex disorder and offers a glimpse into novel treatment strategies that may emerge in the future.

It is now understood that complex changes in neural networks underlie the genesis and perception of tinnitus. This issue begins with a discussion of concepts in this regard that have emerged from animal models, clinical studies, and functional brain imaging. A detailed review of the neurotologist's approach to the patient with tinnitus then follows. The thrust of this issue, however, is in the imaging of the patient with an anatomic, radiologically identifiable, cause of Pulse Synchronous Tinnitus (PST). An overview of the imaging appearances of the more common causes of this condition and a practical approach to the interpretation of imaging studies in the patient with such tinnitus are presented. This review is intended to serve as a handy, practical, and concise summary of the topic. The next few articles discuss in depth the imaging manifestations and endovascular options of some of the more prevalent and sometimes more sinister causes of tinnitus. These include acquired and congenital arterial as well as venous anomalies.

Surgical approaches in the amelioration of tinnitus, with a focus on techniques of sigmoid sinus wall reconstruction, are then discussed in a review that we expect will be of interest to otolaryngologists and neuroradiologists alike. The issue concludes with a review of advanced MR imaging techniques that have demonstrated functional and structural alterations in auditory and nonauditory neural networks in tinnitus sufferers. In summary,

Neuroimag Clin N Am 26 (2016) xiii–xiv
http://dx.doi.org/10.1016/j.nic.2016.03.001
1052-5149/16/$ – see front matter © 2016 Published by Elsevier Inc.

we hope that this issue presents a bird's-eye view of where the field stands today and offers some insights into the work that remains to be done.

First and foremost, we would like to offer our sincere gratitude and appreciation to all the authors that have contributed their excellent work to this issue. We are also grateful to Dr Suresh Mukherji for presenting to us this incredible opportunity and for his guidance. Our heartfelt appreciation for the Elsevier team: John Vassallo, Casey Jackson, Nicole Congleton, and the editorial staff for their help, support, and, most importantly, patience, in the preparation of this issue.

Last, but not least, out personal thanks to our families, for their unending encouragement, patience, and support.

Sincerely,

Prashant Raghavan, MBBS
Division of Neuroradiology
Department of Diagnostic Radiology
and Nuclear Medicine
University of Maryland School of Medicine
Baltimore, MD, USA

Dheeraj Gandhi, MBBS, MD
Division of Interventional Neuroradiology
Department of Diagnostic Radiology
and Nuclear Medicine
University of Maryland School of Medicine
Departments of Neurology and Neurosurgery
University of Maryland School of Medicine
Baltimore, MD, USA

E-mail addresses:
Prashant.raghavan@gmail.com (P. Raghavan)
dgandhi@umm.edu (D. Gandhi)

Neuroscience of Tinnitus

Daniel Ryan, MD[a], Carol A. Bauer, MD[b],*

KEYWORDS

- Tinnitus • Neural networks • Excitotoxicity • Plasticity • Glutamic acid • NMDA • AMPA

KEY POINTS

- Tinnitus is the result of changes in a distributed central neural network following cochlear insult.
- The pathologic conditions producing tinnitus seem to differ at different network levels.
- Understanding and therapeutically addressing tinnitus is complicated by its heterogeneous and distributed pathophysiology.
- Functional brain imaging, histocytochemical analysis, and laboratory and clinical studies have contributed to the current understanding.
- Current and emergent treatment options are targeting pathologic functions revealed by this research.

Tinnitus is the most common chronic auditory disorder. National Health and Nutrition Examination Survey data estimate that approximately 45 million American adults experience tinnitus and 15 million report frequent symptoms.[1 5] Although the definition of tinnitus may affect survey figures, adult prevalence is between 6% and 19%.[6] Hearing loss is the greatest risk factor for developing tinnitus and risk increases with a history of high-level sound exposure earlier in life.[7] The popularity of in-ear and headphone speakers used with recreational sound devices, in addition to the increased average age of the population, and associated cumulative noise exposure, predict a growing health concern.[4,5,8–10] In addition, the US Department of Veterans Affairs estimated that in 2014 approximately 22 million Americans had served in the military,[11] an environment that exposes young adults to potentially damaging high-level sound that places them at increased risk of tinnitus.[12]

Despite the great number people with symptoms, only approximately one-third of those with tinnitus seek care because of its bothersome effects (eg, changes in sleep, disturbed concentration and affect).[4,6] Although there are secondary (objective) forms of tinnitus from organic sources, primary (subjective) tinnitus is an auditory sensation without a corresponding external sound source. It is a consequence of sensorineural hearing loss and central auditory pathway changes.[7] Advances in functional imaging have provided insight into the neural activity in normal and pathologic auditory processing pathways.[13–15] Understanding the neural mechanisms and cellular activity behind the phantom percept may refine treatment and help to develop strategies for prevention and screening.

ANATOMY OF THE AUDITORY PATHWAY

The auditory system is divided grossly into central (upper) and peripheral (lower) divisions.[16] The upper auditory pathway contains the primary auditory cortex (A1), medial geniculate bodies (MGBs), inferior colliculus (IC), superior olivary complex (SOC), and the cochlear nucleus complex (CN).[7] Components of the lower auditory pathway

Disclosure: The authors have nothing to disclose.
[a] Department of Diagnostic Radiology, Southern Illinois University School of Medicine, Memorial Medical Center, 701 North 1st Street, Springfield, IL 62794-9662, USA; [b] Department of Surgery, Southern Illinois University School of Medicine, 301 North 8th Street P.O. Box 19662, Springfield, IL 62794-9662, USA
* Corresponding author.
E-mail address: cbauer@siumed.edu

Neuroimag Clin N Am 26 (2016) 187–196
http://dx.doi.org/10.1016/j.nic.2015.12.001
1052-5149/16/$ – see front matter © 2016 Elsevier Inc. All rights reserved.

are the peripheral auditory structures; namely the pinna, external auditory canal, tympanic membrane, ossicular chain (malleus, incus, and stapes), the cochlea (hair cells, basilar membrane, and spiral ganglion), and the auditory nerve connecting the central and peripheral auditory structures.[7,16] Airborne pressure waves exert a mechanical force on the tympanic membrane that is transmitted via the middle ear ossicles to the cochlea. Mechanical energy and motion of the basilar membrane within the cochlea are transduced by an inner row of hair cells that release neurotransmitter (glutamic acid [Glu]) onto the dendrites of first-order afferent neurons. These neurons form the auditory nerve that enters and forms synapses within the CN in the brainstem.[17]

The cochlea is composed of an osseous labyrinth, a fluid-filled tunneled compartment that courses approximately 2.5 revolutions around its longitudinal axis (the modiolus) within the osseous capsule of temporal bone.[7,16,17] The scala media (cochlear duct) is a compartment enclosed by the membranous labyrinth. It contains a row of inner and 3 rows of outer hair cells laid out along the basilar membrane, along with supporting elements forming the organ of Corti.[17]

The basolateral surfaces of hair cells synapse with spiral ganglion nerve cells.[16,17] Type 1 spiral ganglion cells are large bipolar cells with myelinated fibrils that contact inner hair cells. They represent 90% to 95% of the ganglion cell population. Inner hair cells are also contacted by unmyelinated extensions arising beyond the habenula perforata.[7,16,17] Type 1 spiral ganglion cells are different from type 2 cells, which are smaller, unipolar, and mostly unmyelinated cells that contact outer hair cells.[7,16,17] Inner hair cells are primarily responsible for transducing sound, with the information reaching the brain via type 1 afferents. In contrast, outer hair cells act as modulatory amplifiers, particularly for low-level sound.[16,17]

The spiral ganglion courses through the Rosenthal canal in the central part of the cochlea.[7,16] The cochlear nerve emerges from the pontomedullary junction and courses through the internal acoustic meatus.[16,17] Most auditory nerve fibers synapse within the ipsilateral cochlear nuclei, which are tonotopically organized into anterior ventral cochlear nuclei (AVCN), dorsal cochlear nuclei (DCN), and posterior ventral cochlear nuclei (PVCN) divisions.[7] The AVCN and PVCN process the temporal features of the transmitted signal using membrane capacitance, dendritic filtering, and spatial organization, whereas fusiform cells of the DCN contribute to decoding sound level and directional information.[7,18] Integration of inputs from the somatosensory system in the DCN further improves sound localization.[4,7,13,16] The lateral lemniscus (ie, lemniscal pathway) conveys sound information from the cochlear nucleus rostral to the contralateral IC, and provides input to other nuclei as well.[7,15,16]

Most ascending connections in the IC, comprising the lemniscal pathway, synapse in the centrally located core.[7,12,16] The peripheral shell of the IC, comprising the extralemniscal pathway, receives a mixture of ascending and descending fibers.[4,5,7,13,16] The IC extracts auditory information by integrating both afferent and efferent streams (ie, lower-order and higher-order processes), sending information rostral to the thalamic MGB.[4,5,7,16] The MGB serves as an intelligent router for the auditory pathway to cortex.[7,16] The ventral subdivision of the MGB, a continuation of the lemniscal pathway, is organized tonotopically and uses fast glutamatergic synapses to connect to layers 3 and 4 of the A1.[7,19,20] Much remains to be understood about thalamocortical gating and its role in attention and arousal.

BIOCHEMICAL AND MOLECULAR TRANSDUCTION

The primary and highly preserved excitatory neurotransmitter of the brain, Glu, serves the cochlear hair cell synapses.[7,16,21] Sound-induced deflection of hair cell stereocilia affects mechanosensitive transducer channels at the apex of each hair cell.[16,17] In resting position, the ion channels are partially open, sustaining a moderate depolarizing current in the absence of stimulation.[7,13,17] Deflection of stereocilia results in the release of Glu-containing vesicles at the hair base, and depolarization of primary afferent nerves. In a conserved manner, Glu serves as the primary excitatory neurotransmitter throughout ascending levels of the auditory system.

CENTRAL NETWORK ORGANIZATION

Complex networks exist at many levels in living systems. The most efficient are selected by natural pressures.[22] Mathematical models used to analyze brain networks have shown the utility of so-called small-world organization. Small-world networks are composed of dense, semiregular cell clusters with a high degree of local connectivity and sparse long-range connections.[22–24] This network schema enables distributed, but specialized, processing that is resistant to pathologic degradation. It also provides for efficient communication and the specialized operations necessary to perform multidimensional tasks.[22] Small-world models are increasingly being used to understand human intelligence and to construct models of artificial intelligence.[25]

Although small-world models support efficient local processing, globally the brain is required to parallel process multiple dimensions in real-world tasks. This seems to demand adaptive information transfer between spatially distinct networks, with each contributing to the interpretation of sensory input (ie, perception).[22,24] Using functional MR (fMR) imaging to compare control subjects and people with partial network blockade, Achard and Bullmore[22] in 2007 showed that parallel information processing through a large-scale network maximized cost-efficiency. The human brain seemed to function best when it was able to manipulate information from various spatially and temporally separate processing centers that converge to assign adaptive meaning to sensory information.[23] The cortex is efficient in dynamically recognizing, classifying, and accepting traces of transient neural activity from fluid sources, such as netlets and cortical columns (ie, modules of neurons with emergent properties organized in parametrically classified logistic maps).[25] Model analysis has shown that neural network calculation requirements are reduced in parametrically classified logistic map networks.[25] Understanding brain connectivity (ie, the emergent field of connectomics) may provide an explanation for the computational gain of networks compared with the function of their neural constituents.[23,25]

PERCEPTION AND NONAUDITORY DIMENSIONS OF SOUND

Auditory perception requires the participation of brain areas in addition to those defined as part of the central auditory pathway. Functional blood oxygen level difference (BOLD) and fMR imaging studies in normal-hearing individuals during attention-demanding auditory tasks revealed areas of prefrontal, parietal, cingulate, and insular cortex activity, in addition to those classically defined as auditory areas.[26] Collectively, these areas have been referred to as the global neuronal workspace, and their conjoint activity has been associated with conscious awareness[26,27] (Table 1). These structures have been further divided into a perceptual network, containing the anterior and posterior cingulate cortex and portions of the frontal and parietal cortices, including the precuneus; and a salience network, involving the dorsal-anterior cingulate cortex and the anterior insula[13,28] (see Table 1). Functional imaging studies have shown this global neuronal workspace to be active in tinnitus, when the tinnitus is

Table 1
Global neuronal workspace[56]

Perceptual Network	Salience Network
Anterior cingulate cortex	Dorsal-anterior
Posterior cingulate cortex	cingulate cortex
Precuneus	Anterior insula
Portions of the frontal and parietal cortex	

Data from Guo L. Veteran Population Projection Model 2014. 2014.

perceptible.[26] Furthermore, it has been suggested that neural activity restricted to the auditory system alone (eg, the primary auditory cortex) is insufficient for the conscious experience of either sound or tinnitus.[28,29]

Bothersome tinnitus has been attributed to involvement of emotional networks and rearrangement of their linkage to auditory networks.[26,30,31] Synchronous activity in these two networks might explain identification of delta, alpha, and gamma bands of electroencephalographic (EEG) activity in these locations.[26,32] Magnetoencephalography and EEG studies in subjects with tinnitus have supported a thalamocortical dysrhythmia model whereby changes in electrical activity are characterized by low-frequency delta (≤ 2 Hz) and theta (~ 6 Hz) waves projecting from the auditory thalamus to the auditory cortex that synchronously induce high-frequency gamma oscillations in the auditory cortex; this activity is thought to be part of a normal function comprising auditory attention. Increased thalamic inhibition might subvert the process in tinnitus.[26,33–35] Along with persistent conscious awareness of tinnitus, some patients show involvement of the limbic system (ie, the emotional control network [the anterior cingulate cortex, anterior insula, and amygdala]), which could be derived from plastic recruitment of the hippocampus, parahippocampus, and amygdala.[13,28] Overall, broad regions of cortex, and subcortical structures have been shown to have activity alterations associated with tinnitus.[13] Under nonpathologic circumstances these networks integrate auditory perception with adaptive goal-directed behavior, but in the presence of a persistent internally generated stimulus (tinnitus) their engagement can be disruptive.[7,13,15]

PERIPHERAL AUDITORY SYSTEM RESPONSE TO INSULT

Insult to the cochlea (inner hair cells, outer hair cells, or primary afferent dendrites) may cause a temporary or a permanent disturbance in auditory perception.[7,19] A common insult, high-level sound exposure, can encompass 1 brief exposure, a single very-high-level exposure (blast), or repeated exposures of variable duration and level. All have been documented as potentially damaging spiral ganglion dendrites.[21,36,37] In addition, high-concentration salicylate exposure has been shown to activate cochlear N-methyl-D-aspartate (NMDA) receptors and to decrease auditory nerve activity. Salicylates affect cell membrane integrity, increasing arachidonic acid concentration through cyclooxygenase inhibition, and reversibly inhibiting the motility of prestin, an outer hair cell plasma membrane protein.[4,17,38,39] The effect is to increase hearing thresholds (ie, worsen hearing) and to reduce the cochlear amplification of sound.[7,17,21] Destruction of outer hair cells by other means, even when inner hair cells are preserved, increases hearing thresholds and reduces the auditory signal reaching the central nervous system.[26] There is evidence to suggest that loss of nerve cell dendrites in the cochlea,[40] or loss of their connection to hair cells,[11] may be more important for tinnitus induction than loss of hair cells per se.

CENTRAL DISORDERS OF TINNITUS

A central nervous system response to impaired peripheral sensation is deployed to compensate for the loss.[26,41] The compensatory process can involve a decrease or an increase of tonic inhibition (at different levels in the pathway), upregulation of excitation and spontaneous neural activity, and cortical tonotopic reorganization, with areas devoted to impoverished inputs being reassigned to preserved inputs.[4,7,19,42] Distortion of cortical tonotopic representation is one of the plausible theories proposed to explain tinnitus perception,[4,7] although recent evidence has called its relevance into question.[42] A reciprocal balance of excitation and inhibition seems to characterize central processing, no less so for audition than other systems.[43,44] An imbalance of activity at one level (eg, decreased cochlear activity in specific frequency regions) would be expected to produce a cascade of ascending compensatory effects. Immunocytochemical acetylcholinesterase staining of the primary auditory cortex and its surrounding regions shows input from all sensory modalities in addition to reciprocal connectivity to the cochlea.[45–47] Without an executive center for analysis and integration, the primary function ascribed to cortex, full extraction of signal content would not be possible; for example, in an experimental cat model, primary auditory lobectomy did not compromise orientation and tone discrimination, but the act of approaching the sound to obtain food (ie, the acquired meaning of the sound) was eliminated.[7,48] Because tinnitus is a conscious percept, it is likely that cortical factors contribute to that percept. Furthermore, because cortical networks are integrative, it would be expected that tinnitus would have both cognitive and emotional components and that these overlay factors might vary considerably from one individual to another.[33,49–51] In contrast with the simplicity of the peripheral system, the central auditory system is both plastic and adaptive in response to sound.[33,38] It seems that dysfunction in central networks strengthens and reinforces tinnitus perception and its associated nonauditory distress.[38,52,53]

Variation in cortical, thalamic, and subcortical structures can be measured as periodic field potentials or neurochemical changes, or can be functionally imaged by alterations in neurovascular metabolism or accumulation of neural activity markers. Functional brain imaging has expanded in directions that enable the depiction of brain function in previously unimagined ways.[54] In addition to fMR imaging derived from BOLD measurement, high-resolution voxel-based morphometry (VBM), point-resolved proton spectroscopy, manganese-enhanced MR imaging (MEMRI), as well as PET and single-photon emission tomography have revealed network aspects underlying tinnitus that previously were unknown or purely speculative.[13–15,54–56]

In 2006, Muhlau and colleagues[56] used VBM-MR imaging to show volumetric changes in auditory and nonauditory structures of patients with tinnitus. Specifically, a gray-matter volume loss was observed in the subcallosal area (Zuckerkandl gyrus), an area of the limbic brain with activity correlated with unpleasant emotions.[56–59] This gyrus is not a homogeneous region, but is composed of medial prefrontal, orbitofrontal, and anterior cingulate areas and forms a link between the limbic-affective system and the thalamocortical perceptual system.[4] Other studies have found this region active when listening to aversive sounds and to be modulated by anticipation and perception of pain.[56,57,60,61] The Zuckerkandl gyrus further belongs to the paralimbic ventral striatum, which is critical in forming adaptive behavioral responses to stimuli. Abnormal activity in this region has been found in patients with depressive disorders.[16,56,62,63]

The interconnectivity of the ventral striatum and the cortical subcallosal areas (including the nucleus accumbens [NAc]) allows serotonergic and dopaminergic input to exert their limbic influence on various reward-behavior, avoidance-learning, and emotionally related activities.[64] In this regard the NAc plays a role in pavlovian and instrumental conditioning, together with the dorsal raphe nucleus and other paralimbic regions, and is modulated by serotonergic input to the thalamic reticular nucleus (TRN) and dorsal thalamus.[56,64–68] In the TRN, serotonin excites gamma-aminobutyric acid (GABA)–ergic neurons, which cause inhibition of thalamic sensory relay cells.[4,60] Compared with control animals, rats with NAc lesions show impaired habituation to noise bursts preceded by a warning sound.[64] On this basis it could be hypothesized that conscious awareness of tinnitus is gated by the NAc-TRN system, and its dysfunction might enable the inappropriate transmission of the tinnitus signal to cortex.[4]

The amygdala sends glutamatergic inputs to the NAc that serve as an arousal pathway,[69] and the brainstem raphe nucleus sends serotonergic inputs to the NAc serving as a sleep-cycle pathway.[58,67] The NAc is reciprocally connected with the thalamus, and its TRN connection can inhibit the thalamocortical perceptual pathway.[56,68] Putting this all together, it might be speculated that generalized subcallosal atrophy could derive from emotional, sleep, arousal, habituation, and gating disorders related to tinnitus (Table 2).[56]

MEMRI uses the paramagnetic properties of manganese (Mn^{2+}), which is taken up by active neurons independent of local changes in blood flow or oxygen metabolism, to explore mechanisms underlying tinnitus.[15,70] Mn^{2+} serves as a functional contrast agent capturing neuronal activity through its entry into active neurons through L-type, voltage gated calcium channels (an obligatory link in neural communication via control of neural transmitter release).[15,71–73] Mn^{2+} not only crosses the blood-brain barrier, but when taken up by neurons it remains sequestered for hours to days.[74,75] When used to image tinnitus in rats, relative to matched controls without tinnitus, enhanced activity was shown in the cochlear nucleus (DCN, PVCN, and AVCN), IC, and

paraflocculus (PFL) of the cerebellum.[11,76,77] The increased Mn^{2+} uptake in the cerebellum occurred only in the animals with tinnitus, and was not evident in control animals exposed to an external tinnituslike sound. Furthermore, the increased neural activity was blocked by pretreatment with vigabatrin, a GABA agonist.[15] This result suggests that cerebellar areas undergo a plastic transformation in tinnitus, a process that has been called progressive centralization[78,79] in chronic tinnitus.

Excitatory glutamatergic activity and inhibitory GABAergic activity modulate auditory processing and the balance of these neurotransmitters in auditory and nonauditory pathways is important for adaptive features of audition.[15,80] Treatment of tinnitus with receptor agonists and antagonists alongside functional imaging has helped to show the key consolidative changes made in central auditory pathways as a result of peripheral tinnitus induction.[15] These experimental techniques have enabled the identification of glutamatergic neurons, such as the unipolar brush cell, found within the DCN and PFL that are likely instrumental to the plastic restructuring of auditory pathways triggered by loss of afferent input.[15,81] Application of glutamatergic NMDA-receptor antagonists, such as D(-)-2-amino-5-phosphonopentanoate, in conjunction with functional brain imaging further shows long-term suppression of neural activity and behavioral evidence of tinnitus, which is encouraging for therapeutic efforts directed at tinnitus.[15,76]

CLINICAL THERAPY, EXPERIMENTAL APPROACHES, AND FINDINGS

There is no broadly effective tinnitus treatment, and no standard of care been established. Debate is ongoing about the best approach to correcting the pathophysiologic factors contributing to tinnitus. Contenders include medication directed at either improving inhibitory neurochemical function or inhibiting excitatory function, neuroelectric stimulation (using transcranial electrical or magnetic fields, and cochlear implants), ablation of

Table 2
Parallel nonauditory network structures involved in hearing

Global Neuronal Workspace			
Perceptual Network	Salience Network	Learning Network	Distress Network
Anterior cingulate cortex	Dorsal-anterior	Hippocampus	Anterior Cingulate Cortex
Posterior cingulate	cingulate cortex	Parahippocampus	Anterior insula
Precuneus	Anterior insula	Amygdala	Amygdala
Portions of the frontal and parietal cortex			

auditory or nonauditory brain structures, cognitive/ behavioral counseling therapy, sound exposure, hearing aids, or a combination of approaches.[6] Pharmacologic management of tinnitus in animals and humans has been promising, although a definitive receptor target is still not clear, and addressing multiple targets might be required.[55] Glutamate receptor antagonists reduce damage to the spiral ganglion cells and produce changes in unipolar brush cells that may be useful in both the prevention and modulation of established tinnitus.[15,17,76] In contrast, benzodiazepines (GABA receptor modulators) and gabapentin (chemical analogue of GABA) have shown mixed efficacy when used for tinnitus treatment.[82–85] There are reports of successful reduction of tinnitus loudness and annoyance in clinical trials using a mixed glutamatergic antagonist and GABA agonist, N-acetyl homotaurine (acamprosate)[15,86]; however, replication failure has also be noted.[87]

Surgical treatment of tinnitus historically involved ablative procedures. Most do not provide consistent and reliable relief (and may induce tinnitus). For example, transecting the auditory nerve not only deafens patients but may cause or exacerbate tinnitus.[88] However, ablation of the paraflocculus (a cerebellar area containing a high density of glutamatergic unipolar brush cells) in rats has been reported to eliminate their behavioral evidence of tinnitus, and was also partially effective in preventing tinnitus onset caused by acoustic overstimulation.[70] This study showed that although the paraflocculus is unlikely to be the sole generator of tinnitus, it may be a key component of the compensatory homeostatic network responding to hearing loss and ultimately responsible for tinnitus.[70] The critical interplay between peripheral deafferentation and the central compensatory changes responsible for tinnitus is well shown by the clinical observation of successful treatment using cochlear prosthetic devices. Cochlear implants artificially drive auditory nerve fibers through electrical stimulation of the spiral ganglion. Children and adults with profound hearing loss not improved by conventional hearing aids are candidates for this therapy. It has been reported that cochlear implants not only restored speech discrimination but also greatly reduced or eliminated preexisting tinnitus.[6,17] Dramatically, in one study, the tinnitus percept could be turned on and off by switching the cochlear implant on and off.[89]

In severe cases of debilitating tinnitus, deep brain stimulation of the NAc has been explored as a potential treatment, with mixed results.[4,63,90,91] Similarly, noninvasive extracranial magnetic or electrical fields have been used to stimulate cortical brain areas with the objective of disrupting persistent pathologic neural activity patterns potentially responsible for tinnitus. One variant, transcranial magnetic stimulation has shown some short-term efficacy, but long-term benefits have not been widely confirmed. Limitations include the difficulty of identifying effective target areas, poor field focus, shallow field penetration, and the difficulty of designing well-controlled trials.[4,6] Pharmacologically, stimulating the serotonergic system with selective serotonin reuptake inhibitors (SSRIs) has shown partial efficacy.[92,93] For this therapeutic approach, and perhaps others, there is the issue of causation and comorbidity. Was a therapeutic effect obtained because secondary symptoms were treated rather that the primary symptom, tinnitus? Serotonin depletion has multiple consequences, including reduction in rapid eye movement sleep, anhedonia/depression, and hypersensitivity to sound. Did SSRI therapy address these issues or more directly restore the auditory imbalance responsible for tinnitus.[4,94–97] In addition, research on analogous conditions, such as the chronic pain syndromes, phantom limb pain, and fibromyalgia, may illuminate tinnitus. All 3 conditions may derive from homeostatic overcompensation, and stress seems to similarly exacerbate symptoms.[4,98–101] Treatments designed to improve coping mechanisms, reduce stress, and alleviate anxiety, such as cognitive behavior therapy, have shown promise in reducing the impact of all 3 conditions.

Variable success in managing tinnitus using either direct auditory stimulation or indirect somatic modulation has been shown. In some people tinnitus can be modulated (increased or decreased in loudness) by somatic manipulation of head and neck areas. Somatic modulation is plausible because somatic inputs to the dorsal cochlear nucleus from the trigeminal and cervicospinal pathways are well known.[102] Transcutaneous electrical stimulation of the head and neck has been reported to produce approximately 50% improvement in patients with somatic tinnitus.[6,103] At this time it is unclear whether somatic tinnitus is common or occurs in only a small subset of people with tinnitus. Shore and colleagues[104] hypothesize that auditory deafferentation disinhibits somatic afferents to the dorsal cochlear nucleus. As a result, somatic stimulation inappropriately feeds into the auditory system and produces the tinnitus percept.[105]

Direct stimulation of the auditory pathway through enhanced external sound has been used to treat tinnitus awareness for millennia. Sound therapy may exploit the ubiquitous process of habituation; for example, to background sound.[106,107] It is also possible that increased acoustic stimulation reverses central disorders related to hearing-loss deafferentation.[6] Sound therapy can vary from ear-level devices to environmental free-field sound generators; sound composition can vary from customized low-level frequency bands that match an individual's hearing loss, to broad-band noise, and spectrally modified music. Simple amplification of environmental sound (ie, hearing aids) has also been applied as a tinnitus therapeutic.[6] Controlled trials support the clinical efficacy of all auditory stimulation therapies. For example, bilateral hearing aids improve hearing; reduce the straining-to-hear phenomenon; and reduce, but do not eliminate, tinnitus awareness and annoyance.[6]

SUMMARY

Challenges in addressing the central tinnitus syndrome include the apparent heterogeneity of the patient population, confounding hearing loss, and potential underlying genetic susceptibilities.[4,6] Altogether, loss of inhibition and increased excitation in auditory and nonauditory neural networks likely underlie the central features that follow cochlear damage and are responsible for tinnitus.[4,7] Areas involved in sensory gating or network coordination, such as the subcallosal area and the paraflocculus, have shown their importance in conscious perception of this phantom sound.[56–59] Mechanisms revealed by experimental models can serve as the basis for emergent tinnitus therapies.[6,15,17] Continued advances in the development and understanding of its underlying neural mechanisms will help to address or eliminate this medical problem and possibly related conditions as well.[70]

REFERENCES

1. American tinnitus association. Understanding the facts. 2011. Available at: http://ata.org/understanding-facts. Accessed January 28, 2016.
2. Chang JE, Zeng FG. Tinnitus suppression by electric stimulation of the auditory nerve. Front Syst Neurosci 2012;6:19.
3. Shargorodsky J, Curhan GC, Farwell WR. Prevalence and characteristics of tinnitus among US adults. Am J Med 2010;123(8):711–8.
4. Rauschecker JP, Leaver AM, Muhlau M. Tuning out the noise: limbic auditory interactions of tinnitus. Neuron 2010;66:819–26.
5. Roberts LE, Eggermont JJ, Caspary DM, et al. Ringing ears: the neuroscience of tinnitus. J Neurosci 2010;30(45):14972–9.
6. Bauer CA. Tinnitus. In: Lalwani and Sataloff, editors. Otolaryngology: Head and Neck Surgery. New Delhi (India): Jaypee Brothers; 2014.
7. Brozoski TJ, Bauer CA. Auditory neuronal networks and chronic tinnitus. In: Faingold CL, Blumenfeld H, editors. Neuronal networks in brain function, CNS disorders, and therapeutics. Cambridge (MA): Academic Press; 2014. p. 261–75.
8. Jastreboff PJ. Phantom auditory perception (tinnitus): mechanisms of generation and perception. Neurosci Res 1990;8:221–54.
9. Niskar AS, Kieszak SM, Holmes AE, et al. Estimated prevalence of noise-induced hearing threshold shifts among children 6-19 years of age: the Third National Health and Nutrition Examination Survey, 1988-1994, United States. Pediatrics 2001;108:40–3.
10. Kujawa SG, Liberman MC. Acceleration of age-related hearing loss by early noise exposure: evidence of a misspent youth. J Neurosci 2006;26: 2115–23.
11. Guo L. Veteran population projection model 2014. 2014.
12. Theodoroff SM, Lewis MS, Folmer RL, et al. Hearing impairment and tinnitus: prevalence, risk factors, and outcomes in US service members and veterans deployed to the Iraq and Afghanistan wars. Epidemiol Rev 2015;37:71–85.
13. Song JJ, De Ridder D, Van de Heyning P, et al. Mapping tinnitus-related brain activation: an activation-likelihood estimation metaanalysis of PET studies. J Nucl Med 2012;53:1550–7.
14. Wineland AM, Burton H, Piccirillo J. Functional connectivity networks in nonbothersome tinnitus. Otolaryngol Head Neck Surg 2012;47(5):900–6.
15. Cacace AT, Brozoski T, Berkowitz B, et al. Manganese enhanced magnetic resonance imaging (MEMRI): a powerful new imaging method to study tinnitus. Hear Res 2014;311:49–62.
16. Hudspeth AJ. Hearing. In: Kandel ER, Schwartz JH, Jessell TM, editors. Principles of neural science. New York: McGraw-Hill; 2000. p. 654–711.
17. Raphael Y, Altschuler RA. Structure and innervation of the cochlea. Brain Res Bull 2003;60(5–6):397–422.
18. Arle JE, Kim DO. Neural modeling of intrinsic and spike discharge properties of cochlear nucleus neurons. Biol Cybern 1991;64(4):273–83.
19. Hackett TA, Barkat TR, O'Brien BM, et al. Linking topography to tonotopy in the mouse auditory thalamocortical circuit. J Neurosci 2011; 31(8):2983–95.
20. de la Mothe LA, Blumell S, Kajikawa Y, et al. Thalamic connections of the auditory cortex in marmoset monkeys: core and medial belt regions. J Comp Neurol 2006;496(1):72–96.
21. Sanchez JT, Ghelani S, Otto-Meyer S. From development to disease: diverse functions of NMDA-type

glutamate receptors in the lower auditory pathway. Neuroscience 2015;285:248–59.

22. Achard S, Bullmore E. Efficiency and cost of economical brain functional networks. PLoS Comput Biol 2007;3(2):e17.

23. Abeles M. Corticonics, neural circuits of the cerebral cortex. Cambridge (United Kingdom): Cambridge University Press; 1991.

24. Kaiser M, Hilgetag CC. Nonoptimal component placement, but short processing paths, due to long-distance projections in neural systems. PLoS Comput Biol 2006;2:e95.

25. Farhat NH. Corticonic models of brain mechanisms underlying cognition and intelligence. Phys Life Rev 2007;4:223–52.

26. Eggermont JJ, Roberts LE. The neuroscience of tinnitus: understanding abnormal and normal auditory perception. Front Syst Neurosci 2012; 6(53):5–8.

27. Dehaene S, Changeux JP. Experimental and theoretical approaches to conscious processing. Neuron 2011;70:200–27.

28. De Ridder D, Elgoyhen AB, Romo R, et al. Phantom percepts: tinnitus and pain as persisting aversive memory networks. Proc Natl Acad Sci U S A 2011;108:8075–80.

29. Schlee W, Hartmann T, Langguth B, et al. Abnormal resting-state cortical coupling in chronic tinnitus. BMC Neurosci 2009;10:10–1.

30. Leaver AM, Seydell-Greenwald A, Turesky TK, et al. Cortico-limbic morphology separates tinnitus from tinnitus distress. Front Syst Neurosci 2012;6:21.

31. Vanneste S, Joos K, De Ridder D. Prefrontal cortex based sex differences in tinnitus perception: same tinnitus intensity, same tinnitus distress, different mood. PLoS One 2012;7(2):e31182.

32. Middleton JW, Tzounopoulos T. Imaging the neural correlates of tinnitus: a comparison between animal models and human studies. Front Syst Neurosci 2012;6(35):1–9.

33. Weisz N, Muller S, Schlee W, et al. The neural code of auditory phantom perception. J Neurosci 2007; 27:1479–84.

34. van der Loo E, Gais S, Congedo N, et al. Tinnitus intensity dependent gamma oscillations of the contralateral auditory cortex. PLoS One 2009;4:e7396.

35. De Ridder D, van der Loo E, Vanneste S, et al. Theta-gamma dysrhythmia and auditory phantom perception. J Neurosurg 2011b;114:912–21.

36. Kujawa SG, Liberman MC. Adding insult to injury: cochlear nerve degeneration after "temporary" noise-induced hearing loss. J Neurosci 2009; 29(45):14077–85.

37. Lin HW, Furman AC, Kujawa SG, et al. Primary neural degeneration in the Guinea pig cochlea after reversible noise-induced threshold shift. J Assoc Res Otolaryngol 2011;12:605–16.

38. Guitton MJ. Tinnitus: pathology of synaptic plasticity at the cellular and system levels. Front Syst Neurosci 2012;6(12):215–21.

39. Stolzberg D, Salvi RJ, Allman BL. Salicylate toxicity model of tinnitus. Front Syst Neurosci 2012;6(28): 249–60.

40. Bauer CA, Brozoski TJ, Myers K. Primary afferent dendrite degeneration as a cause of tinnitus. J Neurosci Res 2007;85(7):1489–98.

41. Norena AJ, Farley BJ. Tinnitus-related neural activity: theories of generation, propagation, and centralization. Hear Res 2013;295:161–71.

42. Langers DR, de Kleine E, van Dijk P. Tinnitus does not require macroscopic tonotopic map reorganization. Front Syst Neurosci 2012;6:2.

43. Norena AJ. An integrative model of tinnitus based on a central gain controlling neural sensitivity. Neurosci Biobehav Rev 2011;35(5):1089–109.

44. Knipper M, Van Dijk P, Nunes I, et al. Advances in the neurobiology of hearing disorders: recent developments regarding the basis of tinnitus and hyperacusis. Prog Neurobiol 2013;111:17–33.

45. Kilgard MP, Merzenich MM. Cortical map reorganization enabled by nucleus basalis activity. Science 1998;279(5357):1714–8.

46. Hackett TA. Information flow in the auditory cortical network. Hear Res 2011;271(1–2):133–46.

47. Winer JA, Lee CC. The distributed auditory cortex. Hear Res 2007;229(1–2):3–13.

48. Masterton RB. Role of the mammalian forebrain in hearing. In: Syka J, editor. International symposium on acoustical signal processing in the central auditory system. Prague (Czech Republic): Plenum Press; 1996. p. 1–17.

49. Melcher JR, Sigalvosky IS, Guinan JJ, et al. Lateralized tinnitus studied with functional magnetic resonance imaging: abnormal inferior colliculus activation. J Neurophysiol 2000;83: 1058–72.

50. Eggermont JJ. Central tinnitus. Auris Nasus Larynx 2003;30(Suppl):S7–12.

51. Norena AJ, Eggermont JJ. Enriched acoustic environment after noise trauma reduces hearing loss and prevents cortical map reorganization. J Neurosci 2005;25(3):699–705.

52. Eggermont JJ, Roberts LE. The neuroscience of tinnitus. Trends Neurosci 2004;27(11):676–82.

53. Guitton MJ. Tinnitus and anxiety: more than meets the ears. Curr Psychiatry Rev 2006;2:333–8.

54. Cacace AT, Tasciyan T, Cousins JP. Principles of functional magnetic resonance imaging: application to auditory neuroscience. J Am Acad Audiol 2000;11:239–72.

55. Brozoski T, Odintsov B, Bauer C. Gamma-aminobutyric acid and glutamic acid levels in the auditory pathway of rats with chronic tinnitus: a direct determination using high resolution point-resolved

proton magnetic resonance spectroscopy (H-MRS). Front Syst Neurosci 2012;6:9.

56. Muhlau M, Rauschecker JP, Oestreicher E, et al. Structural brain changes in tinnitus. Cereb Cortex 2006;16:1283–8.

57. Blood AJ, Zatorre RJ, Bermudez P, et al. Emotional responses to pleasant and unpleasant music correlate with activity in paralimbic brain regions. Nat Neurosci 1999;2:382–7.

58. Hyde KL, Zatorre RJ, Evans AC, et al. Structural brain differences in unilateral tinnitus. San Francisco (CA): Organization Human Brain Mapping; 2009.

59. Landgrebe M, Langguth B, Rosengarth K, et al. Structural brain changes in tinnitus: grey matter decrease in auditory and non-auditory brain areas. Neuroimage 2009;46:213–8.

60. Zald DH, Pardo JV. The neural correlates of aversive auditory stimulation. Neuroimage 2002;16:746–53.

61. Ploghaus A, Becerra L, Borras C, et al. Neural circuitry underlying pain modulation: expectation, hypnosis, placebo. Trends Cogn Sci 2003;7:197–200.

62. Drevets WC, Price JL, Simpson JR Jr, et al. Subgenual prefrontal cortex abnormalities in mood disorders. Nature 1997;386:824–7.

63. Mayberg HS, Lozano AM, Voon V, et al. Deep brain stimulation for treatment-resistant depression. Neuron 2005;45:651–60.

64. McCullough LD, Sokolowski JD, Salamone JD. A neurochemical and behavioral investigation of the involvement of nucleus accumbens dopamine in instrumental avoidance. Neuroscience 1993;52:919–25.

65. O'Doherty J, Dayan P, Schultz J, et al. Dissociable roles of ventral and dorsal striatum in instrumental conditioning. Science 2004;304:452–4.

66. Schultz W. Neural coding of basic reward terms of animal learning theory, game theory, microeconomics and behavioral ecology. Curr Opin Neurobiol 2004;14:139–47.

67. Brown P, Molliver ME. Dual serotonin (5-HT) projections to the nucleus accumbens core and shell: relation of the 5-HT transporter to amphetamine-induced neurotoxicity. J Neurosci 2000;20:1952–63.

68. O'Donnell P, Lavin A, Enquist LW, et al. Interconnected parallel circuits between rat nucleus accumbens and thalamus revealed by retrograde transsynaptic transport of pseudorabies virus. J Neurosci 1997;17:2143–67.

69. Koob GF. Neurobiology of addiction. Toward the development of new therapies. Ann N Y Acad Sci 2000;909:170–85.

70. Bauer C, Wisner K, Sybert LT, et al. The cerebellum as a novel tinnitus generator. Hear Res 2013;295:130–9.

71. Inoue T, Majid T, Pautler RG. Manganese enhanced MRI (MEMRI): neurophysiological applications. Rev Neurosci 2011;22(6):675–94.

72. Striessnig J, Bolz HR, Koschak A. Channelopathies in Cav1.1, Cav1.3, and Cav1.4 voltage-gated L-type Ca2+ channels. Pflugers Arch 2010;460(2):361–74.

73. Campbell LW, Hao SY, Thibault O, et al. Aging changes in voltage-gated calcium currents in hippocampal CA1 neurons. J Neurosci 1996;16:6286–95.

74. Koretsky AP, Silva AC. Manganese-enhanced magnetic resonance imaging (MEMRI). NMR Biomed 2004;17(8):527–31.

75. Lee JH, Silva AC, Merkle H, et al. Manganese-enhanced magnetic resonance imaging of mouse brain after systemic administration of MnCl2: dose-dependent and temporal evolution of T1 contrast. Magn Reson Med 2005;53(3):640–8.

76. Brozoski TJ, Wisner KW, Odintsov B, et al. Local NMDA receptor blockade attenuates chronic tinnitus and associated brain activity in an animal model. PLoS One 2013;8(10):e77674.

77. Brozoski TJ, Ciobanu L, Bauer CA. Central neural activity in rats with tinnitus evaluated with manganese-enhanced magnetic resonance imaging (MEMRI). Hear Res 2007;228(1–2):168–79.

78. Mulders WH, Robertson D. Progressive centralization of midbrain hyperactivity after acoustic trauma. Neuroscience 2011;192:753–60.

79. Hickox AE, Liberman MC. Is noise-induced cochlear neuropathy key to the generation of hyperacusis or tinnitus? J Neurophysiol 2014;111(3):552–64.

80. Yang S, Weiner BD, Zhang LS, et al. Homeostatic plasticity drives tinnitus perception in an animal model. Proc Natl Acad Sci U S A 2011;108:14974–9.

81. Mugnaini E, Floris A. The unipolar brush cell: a neglected neuron of the mammalian cerebellar cortex. J Comp Neurol 1994;339(2):174–80.

82. Johnson RM, Brummet R, Schleuning A. Use of alprazolam for relief of tinnitus. A double-blind study. Arch Otolaryngol Head Neck Surg 1993;119:842–5.

83. Jalali MM, Kousha A, Nahavi SE, et al. The effects of alprazolam on tinnitus: a cross-over randomized clinical trial. Med Sci Monit 2009;15:PI55–60.

84. Bauer CA, Brozoski TJ. Effect of gabapentin on the sensation and impact of tinnitus. Laryngoscope 2006;116:675–81.

85. Vanneste S, De Ridder D. The use of alcohol as a moderator for tinnitus-related distress. Brain Topogr 2012;25(1):97–105.

86. Azevedo AA, Figueiredo RR. Tinnitus treatment with acamprosate: double-blind study. Braz J Otorhinolaryngol 2005;71:618–23.

87. Espinosa-Sanchez JM, Heitzmann-Hernandez T, Lopez-Escamez JA. Pharmacotherapy for tinnitus: much ado about nothing. Rev Neurol 2014;59(4):164–74 [in Spanish].

88. House JW, Brackmann DE. Tinnitus: surgical treatment. Ciba Found Symp 1981;85:204–16.

89. Osaki Y, Nishimura H, Takasawa M, et al. Neural mechanism of residual inhibition of tinnitus in cochlear implant users. Neuroreport 2005;16(15): 1625–8.

90. McCracken CB, Grace AA. Nucleus accumbens deep brain stimulation produces region-specific alterations in local field potential oscillations and evoked responses in vivo. J Neurosci 2009;29: 5354–63.

91. Schlaepfer TE, Cohen MX, Frick C, et al. Deep brain stimulation to reward circuitry alleviates anhedonia in refractory major depression. Neuropsychopharmacology 2008;33:368–77.

92. Baldo P, Doree C, Lazzarini R, et al. Antidepressants for patients with tinnitus. Cochrane Database Syst Rev 2006;(4):CD003853.

93. Robinson S. Antidepressants for treatment of tinnitus. Prog Brain Res 2007;166:263–71.

94. Dobie RA. Depression and tinnitus. Otolaryngol Clin North Am 2003;36:383–8.

95. Simpson JJ, Davies WE. A review of evidence in support of a role for 5-HT in the perception of tinnitus. Hear Res 2000;145:1–7.

96. Geyer MA, Vollenweider FX. Serotonin research: contributions to understanding psychoses. Trends Pharmacol Sci 2008;29:445–53.

97. Marriage J, Barnes NM. Is central hyperacusis a symptom of 5-hydroxytryptamine (5-HT) dysfunction? J Laryngol Otol 1995;109:915–21.

98. Flor H, Nikolajsen L, Staehelin Jensen T. Phantom limb pain: a case of maladaptive CNS plasticity? Nat Rev Neurosci 2006;7:873–81.

99. King T, Vera-Portocarrero L, Gutierrez T, et al. Unmasking the tonic-aversive state in neuropathic pain. Nat Neurosci 2009;12:1364–6.

100. Moller AR. Tinnitus and pain. Prog Brain Res 2007; 166:47–53.

101. Folmer RL, Griest SE, Martin WH. Chronic tinnitus as phantom auditory pain. Otolaryngol Head Neck Surg 2001;124:394–400.

102. Shore SE, Zhou J. Somatosensory influence on the cochlear nucleus and beyond. Hear Res 2006; 216–217:90–9.

103. Herraiz C, Toledano A, Diges I. Trans-electrical nerve stimulation (TENS) for somatic tinnitus. Prog Brain Res 2007;166:389–94.

104. Shore SE, Koehler S, Oldakowski M, et al. Dorsal cochlear nucleus responses to somatosensory stimulation are enhanced after noise-induced hearing loss. Eur J Neurosci 2008;27(1):155–68.

105. Dehmel S, Cui YL, Shore SE. Cross-modal interactions of auditory and somatic inputs in the brainstem and midbrain and their imbalance in tinnitus and deafness. Am J Audiol 2008;17(2):S193–209.

106. Hazell JW, Jastreboff PJ. Tinnitus. I: Auditory mechanisms: a model for tinnitus and hearing impairment. J Otolaryngol 1990;19(1):1–5.

107. Weise C, Hesser H, Andersson G, et al. The role of catastrophizing in recent onset tinnitus: its nature and association with tinnitus distress and medical utilization. Int J Audiol 2013;52(3):177–88.

Clinical Evaluation of Tinnitus

Ronna Hertzano, MD, PhD, Taylor B. Teplitzky, BS, David J. Eisenman, MD*

KEYWORDS

• Tinnitus • Subjective tinnitus • Objective tinnitus • Clinical evaluation

KEY POINTS

- The clinical evaluation of patients with tinnitus differs based on whether the tinnitus is subjective or objective.
- Subjective tinnitus is usually associated with a hearing loss, and therefore, the clinical evaluation is focused on an otologic and audiologic evaluation with adjunct imaging/tests as necessary.
- Objective tinnitus is divided into perception of an abnormal somatosound or abnormal perception of a normal somatosound.
- The distinction between these categories is usually possible based on a history, physical examination, and audiogram, leading to directed imaging to identify the underlying abnormality.

INTRODUCTION

Tinnitus Is defined as the perception of sound in the absence of an external sound source. It is further categorized as subjective or objective (Table 1). Subjective tlnnitus may be primary, which may or may not be associated with sensorineural hearing loss, or secondary to a variety of conditions, such as conductive hearing loss, auditory nerve disease, and other conditions. Subjective tinnitus is a purely electrochemical phenomenon and is never audible to an external listener. The site, or more likely sites, of origin of subjective tinnitus likely varies between patients, and identification of potential sites is a subject of intense research efforts. Objective tinnitus is the perception of an actual, mechanical somatosound. Depending on the nature and location of the source, as well as the diligence of the examiner, it may be audible to an objective listener. The most common objective tinnitus arises from self-perception of a vascular somatosound, a so-called pulsatile, or more properly pulse-synchronous, tinnitus.[1] Objective tinnitus can be caused by the perception of an abnormal somatosound, that is, abnormal sound production, or a heightened auditory sensitivity to a normal somatosound, that is, abnormal sound perception. Examples of the former include an arterial-venous malformation or a sigmoid sinus diverticulum, and examples of the latter include a variety of conditions resulting in conductive hearing loss or a pathologic third mobile window of the otic capsule.

The clinical evaluation of the patient with tinnitus is focused on gathering the necessary information to determine the type and cause of this disorder and to formulate thereby an appropriate treatment approach. Although the articles in this issue are focused primarily on objective, pulse-synchronous tinnitus, nonrhythmic, subjective tinnitus is far more common, representing more than 90% of all patients with a chief complaint of tinnitus.[2] Subjective tinnitus, although rarely treated by surgical intervention, also warrants a thorough neurotologic evaluation, sometimes supplemented by diagnostic imaging, with a goal of identifying potentially worrisome or treatable causes. Importantly, because of

The authors have nothing to disclose.
Department of Otorhinolaryngology–Head and Neck Surgery, University of Maryland School of Medicine, 16 South Eutaw Street, Suite 500, Baltimore, MD 21201, USA
* Corresponding author.
E-mail address: deisenman@smail.umaryland.edu

Neuroimag Clin N Am 26 (2016) 197–205
http://dx.doi.org/10.1016/j.nic.2015.12.004
1052-5149/16/$ – see front matter © 2016 Elsevier Inc. All rights reserved.

Table 1
Classification of tinnitus

	Type of Tinnitus	Examples
Objective	Perception of an abnormal somatosound	• Nonvascular causes ○ Palatal myoclonus ○ Tensor tympani/stapedial myoclonus ○ Patulous eustachian tube ○ Idiopathic intracranial hypertension • Vascular ○ Arterial: carotid bruit, atrioventricular malformation, tumors (See Miller TR, Serulle Y, GandhiD: Arterial Abnormalities Leading to Tinnitus, in this issue.) ○ Venous: Sigmoid sinus wall anomalies, transverse sinus stenosis (see Reardon MA, Raghavan P: Venous Abnormalities Leading to Tinnitus: Imaging Evaluation, in this issue.)
	Abnormal perception of a normal somatosound	• Conductive hearing loss • Otic capsule anomalies (eg, SSCD)
Subjective	Primary	• Secondary to a sensorineural hearing loss • Idiopathic (see Hui FK, Abruzzo T, Ansari SA: Endo-vascular Interventions for Idiopathic Intracranial Hypertension and Venous Tinnitus: New Horizons: Imaging Evaluation, in this issue.)
	Secondary	• Conductive hearing loss (eg, middle ear disease, tympanic membrane perforation, otosclerosis, cerumen impaction, eustachian tube dysfunction) • Inner ear disease (eg, Meniere disease) • Otic capsule anomalies (eg, SSCD) • Auditory nerve disease (eg, vestibular schwannoma) • Somatic tinnitus (related to temporomandibular joint dysfunction, cervical dysfunction, or other sensory stimuli) • Associated with affective or other disorders

the high prevalence of subjective tinnitus (30% in individuals 55–99 years old[3]), many patients will report more than one type of tinnitus, each requiring the appropriate clinical evaluation.

CLINICAL EVALUATION OF TINNITUS
Basic Otologic Evaluation

History
The clinical evaluation of tinnitus begins with a complete history and a head and neck examination. A conceptual challenge in the evaluation of tinnitus consists of the categorization of tinnitus into objective and subjective. Historically, objective tinnitus was considered one that a clinician can also hear as part of the medical evaluation. However, as noted earlier, this is not always the case, and true mechanical somatosounds may not be audible even to the most diligent listener. A more useful clinical definition of objective tinnitus is that which, based on its clinical characteristics, is thought to arise from perception of an actual, mechanical somatosound. Therefore, the first step in the evaluation of tinnitus is a clear characterization of the chief complaint and specifically

the acoustic nature of the tinnitus (**Fig. 1**). Based on the patient's description, it is almost always possible to determine if the tinnitus is a result of a somatosound. The most common somatosounds are typically described as "a heartbeat in the ear," "a pulsating hum," "a whooshing sound," "clicking," or "fluttering," depending on their source. Vascular somatosounds often increase in loudness and rate with physical activity and may be modulated by compression or rotation of the neck or other head movements. In contrast, subjective tinnitus is usually described as a continuous high-pitched beep, ringing, cricketlike sound, roaring, ocean noise, or humming. Subjective tinnitus is less likely to be affected by changes in head position or pressure on the neck, although a subgroup of subjective tinnitus sufferers—those

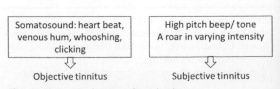

Fig. 1. First step in assessing tinnitus.

with a so-called somatic tinnitus—may be able to alter the quality of the sound, or even abolish it, with certain actions, commonly jaw clenching or thrusting, or occipital pressure. Both types of tinnitus tend to be more bothersome in a quiet acoustic environment, although some patients with subjective tinnitus have worsening symptoms in the presence of sound.

In addition to categorizing the tinnitus as subjective or objective based on the acoustic characteristics and pattern, additional questioning should determine laterality; duration of symptoms; persistence (constant vs intermittent); exacerbating and alleviating factors, including whether the tinnitus is worse in a noisy or quiet environment, with or following certain activities, dietary factors, or seasonal or daily fluctuations. It is critically important to distinguish whether the tinnitus is bothersome or intrusive, because this factor will influence the treatment options to be offered. Patients should be asked about associated symptoms, such as subjective hearing loss, disequilibrium or vertigo, autophony (hearing their own voice in their ear), otalgia, otorrhea, aural fullness or pressure, and blurry vision. The otologic history should include questions about childhood ear infections, noise exposure, known otologic disease, or trauma. The general past medical history should include questions directed at detecting a history of high blood pressure, vascular malformations, carotid stenosis and atherosclerotic disease, stroke or transient ischemic attacks, rapid weight gain or loss, migraine and other types of headache, visual changes, anemia, and thyroid function. Other pertinent information includes a previous history of cancer or chemotherapy (which may also be associated with weight loss), medications, and family history of hearing loss, ear disease, or vestibular schwannoma.

Physical examination
The physical examination consists of a complete head and neck examination, supplemented by a neurotologic examination that includes evaluation of eye movements for nystagmus, complete assessment of cranial nerve function, and a careful otoscopic examination. Auscultation in multiple locations over the mastoid process and over the carotid arteries is critical in patients complaining of perception of a pulse-synchronous sound. If the examiner can perceive the sound themselves, this increases the likelihood that a cause will be identified, and it also provides the patient with much needed reassurance that there is an objectively identifiable correlate for their subjective perception. The authors prefer to use a digital stethoscope (Thinklabs One; Thinklabs Medical LLC, Quebec, Centennial, CO, USA www.thinklabs.com) with noise-cancellation headphones for the greatest sensitivity, although conventional electronic stethoscopes or traditional acoustic stethoscopes are also useful. In addition, a Toynbee tube can be used for auscultation within the external auditory canal.

Once tinnitus is classified as objective or subjective based on the history and physical examination, it is important to assess the patient's hearing. Specifically, it is critical to determine whether there is an associated hearing loss, and if so, whether it is conductive or sensorineural. Hearing is the auditory sensation of environmental movement. Sound is compression and rarefaction of air. Sound waves are transmitted through the external auditory canal to the lateral surface of the tympanic membrane. The tympanic membrane is the lateral border of the middle ear. The sensory cells of hearing, the hair cells, are located in the cochlea, which is a fluid-filled structure in the inner ear. The middle ear is an air-filled chamber that serves as an impedance matching system between the air of the external auditory canal and the fluid of the inner ear. The ability of sound to overcome the impedance mismatch between air and fluid and propagate to the hair cells depends in part on the large vibratory surface area of the tympanic membrane in comparison to the small surface area of the stapes footplate as well as the elasticity of the tympanic membrane and the lever arms of the ossicular chain.[4] Impedance matching also requires equalization of pressure between the middle ear and external auditory canal. Middle ear pressure equilibrates via the eustachian tube, a bony and cartilaginous canal that opens in the nasopharynx, where it is exposed to ambient air pressure.

Processes that disrupt the sound conduction mechanism can lead to conductive hearing loss. These processes can be disorders that prevent sound from reaching the tympanic membrane such as cerumen impaction or otitis externa, violate tympanic membrane integrity such as a perforation, disrupt the ossicular chain such as otosclerosis, cholesteatoma, or necrosis, and/or alter middle ear aeration such as the various forms of eustachian tube dysfunction. Individuals with a conductive hearing loss tend to have a heightened sensation of somatosounds, such that sounds normally produced in the body but typically masked by ambient noise are now audible; this is commonly observed in nonpathologic settings when an individual perceives their heartbeat in the ear resting on a pillow while trying to fall asleep. A second process that can result in a heightened sensation of somatosounds is an otic capsule third mobile window syndrome, most commonly seen with superior semicircular canal dehiscence (SSCD) syndrome. Although third mobile windows can produce a sensorineural hearing loss, they can also result in better than normal bone conduction with a conductive hyperacusis, usually in the lower frequencies.[5]

Careful examination for evidence of abnormality that can result in a conductive hearing loss is a critical part of the evaluation of the patient with tinnitus. In addition to otoscopy, this includes tuning fork tests. The Weber and Rinne tests can suggest a sensorineural or conductive hearing loss. Auditory perception of a tuning fork placed on the lateral malleolus, the so-called lateral malleolar sign, can suggest a third mobile window syndrome or other conductive hyperacusis. Before performing the otologic examination, cerumen should be meticulously removed to allow proper visualization of the entire tympanic membrane. Although sensorineural hearing loss is commonly associated with subjective tinnitus, conductive hearing loss can also result in an identical perception. Therefore, evaluation of a patient with tinnitus is not complete without comprehensive audiometry.

Audiogram
Every patient evaluated for tinnitus should have a comprehensive audiogram. This examination consists of several components: (1) Measurement of pure tone thresholds: Assessment of the threshold at which the patient is able to detect pure tones varying in frequency from 250 to 8000 Hz. This assessment is a behavioral test of a psychophysical measure, because it depends on the patient's report of the minimal intensity at which a sound was audible. Sounds are presented via air (eg, headphones) and bone conduction (using a bone transducer). If the detection of sound is better when the sound is introduced via bone than via air, a so-called air-bone gap conductive abnormality is implied and quantified. Normal hearing is accepted as a threshold of less than 15 dB at all frequencies tested for both ears. Most of the population starts to lose sensitivity to higher frequencies at puberty, and this progresses with age. Any hearing loss can be associated with subjective tinnitus. (2) Speech audiometry: This determines both the minimal intensity at which spoken words (spondees) can be repeated 50% of the time (speech reception threshold), and the percentage of words that the patient repeats correctly when presented at a suprathreshold stimulus (word recognition score). Beyond the functional significance of the tests, the results can suggest a retrocochlear abnormality, such as a vestibular schwanomma (a cause of subjective hearing loss), when the word recognition is decreased

out of proportion to an increase the pure tone thresholds. (3) Acoustic reflex testing: This measures reflex contraction of the stapedius muscle in response to an ipsilateral or contralateral acoustic stimulus. The reflex arc passes through the eighth nerve, auditory and facial nuclei, and facial nerve. This acoustic reflex testing is an objective and quantitative test and can therefore sometimes be helpful in detecting malingerers with inconsistent responses on behavioral tests. Acoustic reflexes are often lost with retrocochlear abnormality, due to abnormality in the afferent limb, and at a very low threshold with most middle ear conductive abnormality, due to an absence of or inability to record the response. However, in a patient with air-bone gaps on pure tone testing, and intact acoustic reflexes, a third mobile window syndrome should be suspected. (4) Impedance testing: This test is another mechanical measure of middle ear function and assesses movement of the tympanic membrane and the pressure in the middle ear cleft, providing objective and quantitative information on the function of the eustachian tube. Acoustic reflex and impedance testing are together referred to as measures of immittance.

At the completion of the history, physical examination, and audiogram, the clinician should be able to determine if the tinnitus is likely objective or subjective and proceed with further evaluation, as needed, using a disease-specific approach (**Table 2**).

Evaluation of subjective tinnitus
The most common cause of subjective tinnitus is sensorineural hearing loss. Subjective tinnitus associated with a sensorineural hearing loss is most frequently described as a high-frequency, continuous tone that is constant or intermittent. It is typically more noticeable in a quiet environment, although some patients will have tinnitus that transiently intensifies during or after exposure to louder sounds.

If this type of subjective tinnitus lateralizes to one ear, is associated with asymmetric hearing loss or other focal neurologic anomalies, or has an abrupt onset in association with a sudden loss in hearing or balance, diagnostic imaging to exclude a worrisome retrocochlear lesion is indicated.[6] The definition of asymmetric sensorineural hearing loss as a guideline for obtaining further evaluation with imaging has been a subject of debate. Commonly used criteria are a 10-dB difference in hearing thresholds in 3 consecutive frequencies, 15 dB in 2 consecutive frequencies, 15 dB at 3000 Hz, or a difference of 15% in the word recognition scores between the 2 ears.[7]

Table 2
Advance diagnostic testing in the evaluation of tinnitus

Type of Tinnitus	Advanced Diagnostic Testing
Subjective tinnitus	
With sensorineural hearing loss	
Tinnitus is symmetric and hearing loss is symmetric	No further evaluation required
Tinnitus or hearing loss are asymmetric	MR imaging of the brain and IAC with and without gadolinium to rule out retrocochlear abnormality
With a conductive hearing loss	
Suspected ossicular abnormality	CT scan of the temporal bones without contrast on a case-specific basis
Bilateral eustachian tube dysfunction	Flexible endoscopic examination of the nasopharynx
Unilateral eustachian tube dysfunction	Flexible endoscopic examination of the nasopharynx +/− additional imaging (CT scan or MR imaging) and biopsy
With inner ear disease	
Meniere disease	This is a clinical diagnosis. MR imaging of the brain and IAC with and without contrast to rule out retrocochlear abnormality
With otic capsule anomalies	
Superior semicircular canal dehiscence	High-resolution CT scan of the temporal bones formatted at the axis of the superior semicircular canal. May obtain adjunct physiologic tests (eg, VEMP)
Objective tinnitus	
Perception of an abnormal somatosound—nonvascular	
Palatal myoclonus	MR imaging of the brain to rule out a brainstem or cerebellar lesion
Tensor tympani/stapedial myoclonus	MR imaging of the brain to rule out a central lesion
Patulous eustachian tube	Flexible endoscopic examination of the nasopharynx No additional imaging is required
Perception of an abnormal somatosound: vascular	1. Contrast-enhanced high-resolution CT scan of the temporal bones with delayed imaging to show the dural venous sinuses. If no abnormality is identified, consider digital subtraction angiography. 2. Carotid duplex ultrasound and/or MR angiography for suspected carotid artery abnormality.

When tinnitus is asymmetric or associated with an asymmetric hearing loss, the imaging of choice is an MR imaging of the brain and internal auditory canals (IACs), with and without gadolinium to rule out retrocochlear abnormality. A recent meta-analysis suggests that auditory brainstem response testing can be used as an alternative in select cases.[8] On the other hand, when a subjective, nonlateralizing primary tinnitus is associated with symmetric hearing, and in the absence of any other neurologic findings, additional imaging is not necessary. In select cases, genetic testing may be considered to determine the cause of the hearing loss.[9]

Subjective tinnitus may be considered primary when there is no other associated cause or when

it is associated with sensorineural hearing loss. It is important to remember that the standard audiogram measures hearing only up to 8000 Hz, while many people can hear up to 20,000 Hz. It is possible to test the hearing in the frequencies between 8000 and 20,000 Hz (also known as an ultra-high-frequency audiogram). This measure can be useful in the evaluation of tinnitus as a result of an exposure to ototoxic agents (eg, Cisplatin chemotherapy). However, these tests otherwise currently have limited clinical utility.

Subjective tinnitus secondary to conductive hearing loss requires additional, directed neurotologic evaluation. Ossicular chain disorders, such as otosclerosis, ossicular necrosis from chronic otitis media, and ossicular dislocation from temporal bone trauma, can be evaluated with a high-resolution computed tomographic (CT) scan of the temporal bones. These disorders are often suspected from the history, physical examination, and specific characteristics of the audiogram. Ossicular dislocation or necrosis is often detectable with high-resolution temporal bone CT, and although imaging is not necessary, it can increase the surgeon's confidence in counseling the patient about the cause of disease, anticipated surgical outcomes, and risks. In otosclerosis, high-resolution CT scan has a sensitivity of greater than 50% in identifying pathologic demineralization of the otic capsule.[10] Conductive hearing loss as a result of a cholesteatoma is often similarly evaluated with a high-resolution noncontrast CT scan of temporal bones. In select cases or when recurrent cholesteatoma is suspected in a region not assessable with otoscopy, MR imaging of the temporal bones with diffusion-weighted imaging is performed. Tinnitus secondary to eustachian tube dysfunction is primarily a diagnosis of exclusion. There are no completely reliable tests of eustachian tube function, and even in the presence of eustachian tube dysfunction as suggested by negative middle ear pressure on immittance testing, other causes still need to be excluded. Unilateral eustachian tube dysfunction in an adult, specifically if this is associated with a unilateral conductive hearing loss and serous otitis media, must always be thoroughly evaluated to exclude nasopharyngeal abnormality. An office, flexible fiberoptic examination and/or a CT scan usually suffices, although MR imaging can be used. Biopsy should be considered on a case-specific basis if the initial diagnostic evaluation has not sufficiently excluded the possibility of a nasopharyngeal neoplasm.

Subjective tinnitus secondary to inner ear disease occurs commonly from Meniere disease and other forms of endolymphatic hydrops such as cochlear hydrops. Meniere disease is thought to result from pressure changes in the endolymph and is characterized by episodes of vertigo lasting more than 20 minutes and less than 24 hours with a sensorineural hearing loss measured at least once in the affected ear.[11] Patients with Meniere disease often complain of a baseline high-pitched tinnitus associated with a sensorineural hearing loss, and a roaring or humming tinnitus that increases in intensity before or during their episodes of vertigo. Meniere disease is a clinical diagnosis. Many patients with Meniere also suffer from migraine,[12] and the diagnosis of vestibular migraine can often be difficult to distinguish from Meniere itself. Complete audiometry is probably the most useful test for distinguishing the 2

pathologic entities.[13] The International Headache Society recently adopted new terminology and diagnostic criteria for vestibular migraine, although their clinical utility has yet to be proven.[14] MR imaging of the brain and IAC with and without contrast is indicated as part of the initial evaluation of patients with suspected Meniere disease. Other specialized tests, such as electrocochleography and vestibular evoked myogenic potentials (VEMP), are sometimes helpful in diagnosing Meniere disease as well.

Subjective tinnitus secondary to otic capsule anomalies refers most commonly to third mobile window abnormalities. The bony labyrinth is the densest bone in the body and normally has only 2 mobile regions: the oval window in which the stapes articulates, and the round window that is sealed by the soft tissue round window membrane. A third window abnormality implies an additional opening of the bony otic capsule, most commonly over the superior semicircular canal leading to a SSCD syndrome. The typical clinical features of SSCD are (a) low-frequency conductive hearing loss; (b) a supranormal bone conductive resulting in an unusual ability to hear somatosounds; and (c) pressure-induced vertigo.[15] Affected patients often report hearing their own body sounds such as their footsteps and eye movements, and autophony, that is, hearing their own voice in their ear when they speak. They can also experience high-frequency tinnitus secondary to the hearing loss as well as pulse synchronous tinnitus from hearing their heartbeat in the affected ears. Clinical testing includes a lateral malleolar test (considered positive when vibrations from a tuning fork placed on the lateral malleolus are heard in the affected ear), sound/pressure-induced nystagmus, and a characteristic audiogram as described above. Imaging consists of a high-resolution CT scan of the temporal bones formatted in the plane of the superior semicircular canal. Finally, not all people with SSCD are symptomatic. Therefore, patients with a suspected abnormality as a result of an SSCD are further evaluated with neurophysiologic testing. This testing includes measurement of VEMP, in which cervical or ocular movements are recorded in response to sound stimuli, in a reflex arc mediated by the saccule or utricle.[16–18] Patients with SSCD that could result in symptoms tend to have abnormally low thresholds and high amplitudes in this test. Electrocochleography has also been shown to be useful in diagnosis of SSCD, and for intraoperative confirmation of adequate canal occlusion.[19,20]

Evaluation of objective tinnitus The evaluation of objective tinnitus consists of first determining whether the somatosound is heard due to an abnormally heightened perception or if it is a consequence of abnormal sound production. Abnormal sound perception is commonly caused by conductive hearing loss or third mobile window syndromes, both of which were reviewed earlier, although it can also be seen with eustachian tube dysfunction.

Patulous eustachian tube Patulous eustachian tube is a condition whereby the eustachian tube exhibits abnormal and sometimes constant patency.[21] Causes for this condition include atrophy of the peritubal fat tissue (which can be seen in patients with rapid weight loss such as those undergoing treatment for malignancy) with loss of venous tone of the pterygoid venous plexus, and also with peritubal musculature dysfunction. It may also be associated with pregnancy. Each of these leads to a concave defect in the tubal valve's anterolateral wall.[22] Common symptoms associated with patulous eustachian tube include self-perception of both one's voice (autophony) and breathing (audible respirations) and aural fullness. Evaluation of patients with patulous eustachian tube includes otoscopy, which often reveals a tympanic membrane that moves synchronously with respiration.[23] Movement may be enhanced with occlusion of one nostril. Patients should have an audiogram and tympanometry. Imaging is not required.

Palatal myoclonus Palatal myoclonus occurs when the soft palate experiences pathologic recurrent contractions.[24] There are 2 main types of palatal myoclonus. Symptomatic palatal myoclonus is often due to a localized lesion in the brainstem or upper cerebellar peduncle (the dentato-rubro-olivary triangle of Guillian and Mollaret). Essential palatal myoclonus occurs when no discrete lesion can be identified. Objective tinnitus is more commonly a complaint of patients with essential, versus symptomatic, palatal myoclonus.[25] In this case, the tinnitus is often of a clicking quality. Evaluation of patients with palatal myoclonus includes physical examination to assess aberrant movement of the soft palate. In addition, patients should have a full audiologicaassessment to rule out a middle ear cause. Patients should be evaluated with an MR imaging of the brain and brainstem to assess for a localized lesion and rule out symptomatic palatal myoclonus.

Tensor tympani/stapedial myoclonus Tinnitus from middle ear myoclonus is due to aberrant contraction of the tensor tympani or the stapedius muscles causing movement of the tympanic membrane in the absence of external sound stimulation.[26] Contraction of the tensor tympani often results in tinnitus characterized by clicking, whereas contraction of the stapedius is often perceived as buzzing, although this distinction is insufficiently consistent to be of clinical utility. Although the underlying cause of middle ear myoclonus has not yet been fully elucidated, Park and colleagues[26] postulate it is due to loud noise exposure in combination with stress. Dehydration and electrolyte abnormalities may also play a role. In addition, myoclonic movements are a subtype of segmental myoclonus that involves muscles innervated by specific areas of the brainstem. Park and colleagues[26] therefore propose causes of segmental myoclonus, including infectious, vascular, traumatic, demyelinating, lesions, and idiopathic, may also result in middle ear myoclonus. Evaluation of patients with middle ear myoclonus includes otoscopy and an impedance audiogram, which includes tympanogram, stapedial reflex, acoustic reflex decay, and static compliance. Observation of the tympanic membrane while the patient is exposed to noise stimuli may also be of benefit. Assessment of blood chemistries can be of value in selected patients. In addition, diagnostic MR Imaging of the brain to assess for central lesions is important, particularly in refractory cases.

Tinnitus from an abnormal arterial or venous somatosound Typically, an arterial pulse synchronous tinnitus will not change in intensity as a result of light pressure on the ipsilateral of the neck; however, this is insufficiently reliable to be used as an isolated diagnostic criterion. The clinician should listen for a carotid bruit and if present refer the patient for carotid ultrasound. Neoplasms of the middle ear and jugular foramen can often be seen otoscopically or present with focal neurologic findings such as lower cranial nerve dysfunction. If a middle ear paraganglioma (glomus tympanicum) can be seen circumferentially on otoscopy, further imaging is not necessary. If it extends below the inferior annular rim of the tympanic membrane, diagnostic CT is needed to assess the intratemporal extent. If there is jugular foramen involvement or extratemporal extension, diagnostic MR imaging of the brain with thin cuts through the temporal bone with and without contrast is the imaging modality of choice. If the nature of a jugular foramen lesion is uncertain with the initial diagnostic evaluation, angiography is helpful in achieving greater diagnostic specificity. Otherwise, angiography is usually reserved for immediate preoperative embolization of vascular lesions.

Venous pulse synchronous tinnitus commonly results from sigmoid sinus wall anomalies (dehiscence, diverticulum, or ectasia), transverse sinus stenosis, idiopathic intracranial hypertension, a high and dehiscent jugular bulb or jugular diverticulum, or condylar vein abnormalities. Importantly, sigmoid sinus wall anomalies, transverse sinus stenosis, and idiopathic intracranial hypertension are frequent comorbidities, and the clinical evaluation should be tailored to assess all 3 abnormalities when any one is suspected.[27,28] Venous pulse synchronous tinnitus typically decreases with light ipsilateral pressure on the neck, sufficient to decrease flow in the jugular vein but not the carotid artery, and it sometimes increases with contralateral pressure. The associated bruit can sometimes be heard with auscultation over the mastoid or in the external auditory canal, but in the authors' experience, more often than not the sound is not objectively audible. Although the algorithm for diagnostic imaging is controversial, the authors favor initial testing with a modified high-resolution CT angiogram of the temporal bones. Image acquisition is with bone windows, and the contrast injection is delayed to ensure venous enhancement. (See Raghavan P, Steven A, Gandhi D: Advanced Neuroimaging of Tinnitus, in this issue.) This protocol allows for assessment of subtle bony abnormalities, such as sigmoid sinus or SSCD, sigmoid sinus diverticulum and transverse sinus stenosis, as well as many of the indirect signs of an acquired dural vascular lesion such as asymmetric arterial feeding vessels, "shaggy" appearance of a dural venous sinus, transcalvarial venous channels, asymmetric venous collaterals, and abnormal size and number of cortical veins.[29] Although the delayed injection prohibits assessment of early venous filling, asymmetric venous attenuation may still be identified if present. Depending on the clinical and imaging findings, further diagnostic evaluation for idiopathic intracranial hypertension with neuro-ophthalmologic examination and lumbar puncture may be considered. If the modified CT angiogram is unrevealing, digital subtraction angiography is considered. Direct communication between the interventional radiologist and referring neurotologist or other clinician is important to ensure that all suspected abnormality, both arterial and venous, is assessed with the catheter-based procedure.

SUMMARY

The clinical evaluation of the patient with tinnitus can be divided into 3 conceptual stages. The first consists of the history, which for most patients will allow for a distinction between objective and subjective tinnitus. Next, in combination with the history, the physical examination and comprehensive audiogram will lead to the determination if for objective tinnitus there is abnormally heightened sound perception or abnormal sound production. For subjective tinnitus, this will distinguish between primary and secondary. At this point, the practicing physician will have sufficient information to decide about proceeding with further specialized testing to identify the underlying pathologic cause.

REFERENCES

1. Mattox DE, Hudgins P. Algorithm for evaluation of pulsatile tinnitus. Acta Otolaryngol 2008;128:427–31.
2. Stouffer JL, Tyler RS. Characterization of tinnitus by tinnitus patients. J Speech Hear Disord 1990;55:439–53.
3. Sindhusake D, Mitchell P, Newall P, et al. Prevalence and characteristics of tinnitus in older adults: the Blue Mountains hearing study. Int J Audiol 2003;42:289–94.
4. Merchant SN, Nadol JB. Schuknecht's pathology of the ear. 3rd edition. Shelton (CT): People's Medical Publishing House; 2010. p. 98–104.
5. Merchant SN, Rosowski JJ. Conductive hearing loss caused by third-window lesions of the inner ear. Otol Neurotol 2008;29:282–9.
6. Tunkel DE, Bauer CA, Sun GH, et al. Clinical practice guideline: tinnitus. Otolaryngol Head Neck Surg 2014;151:S1–40.
7. Ahsan SF, Standring R, Osborn DA, et al. Clinical predictors of abnormal magnetic resonance imaging findings in patients with asymmetric sensorineural hearing loss. JAMA Otolaryngol Head Neck Surg 2015;141:451–6.
8. Koors PD, Thacker LR, Coelho DH. ABR in the diagnosis of vestibular schwannomas: a meta-analysis. Am J Otolaryngol 2013;34:195–204.
9. Shearer AE, Black-Ziegelbein EA, Hildebrand MS, et al. Advancing genetic testing for deafness with genomic technology. J Med Genet 2013;50:627–34.
10. Karosi T, Csomor P, Sziklai I. The value of HRCT in stapes fixations corresponding to hearing thresholds and histologic findings. Otol Neurotol 2012;33:1300–7.
11. Committee on hearing and equilibrium guidelines for the diagnosis and evaluation of therapy in Meniere's disease. American Academy of Otolaryngology-Head and Neck Foundation, Inc. Otolaryngol Head Neck Surg 1995;113:181–5.
12. Ishiyama G, Lopez IA, Sepahdari AR, et al. Meniere's disease: histopathology, cytochemistry, and imaging. Ann N Y Acad Sci 2015;1343:49–57.
13. Battista RA. Audiometric findings of patients with migraine-associated dizziness. Otol Neurotol 2004;25:987–92.
14. Headache Classification Committee of the International Headache Society (IHS). The International

Classification of Headache Disorders, 3rd edition (beta version). Cephalalgia 2013;33:629–808.

15. Minor LB. Clinical manifestations of superior semicircular canal dehiscence. Laryngoscope 2005;115:1717–27.

16. Dennis DL, Govender S, Colebatch JG. Properties of cervical and ocular vestibular evoked myogenic potentials (cVEMPs and oVEMPs) evoked by 500 Hz and 100 Hz bone vibration at the mastoid. Clin Neurophysiol 2016;127:848–57.

17. Milojcic R, Guinan JJ Jr, Rauch SD, et al. Vestibular evoked myogenic potentials in patients with superior semicircular canal dehiscence. Otol Neurotol 2013;34:360–7.

18. Colebatch JG, Halmagyi GM, Skuse NF. Myogenic potentials generated by a click-evoked vestibulocollic reflex. J Neurol Neurosurg Psychiatr 1994;57:190–7.

19. Park JH, Lee SY, Song JJ, et al. Electrocochleographic findings in superior canal dehiscence syndrome. Hear Res 2015;323:61–7.

20. Adams ME, Kileny PR, Telian SA, et al. Electrocochleography as a diagnostic and intraoperative adjunct in superior semicircular canal dehiscence syndrome. Otol Neurotol 2011;32:1506–12.

21. Hussein AA, Adams AS, Turner JH. Surgical management of Patulous Eustachian tube: a systematic review. Laryngoscope 2015;125:2193–8.

22. Poe DS. Diagnosis and management of the patulous eustachian tube. Otol Neurotol 2007;28:668–77.

23. Doherty JK, Slattery WH 3rd. Autologous fat grafting for the refractory patulous eustachian tube. Otolaryngol Head Neck Surg 2003;128:88–91.

24. Deuschl G, Wilms H. Clinical spectrum and physiology of palatal tremor. Mov Disord 2002;17(Suppl 2):S63–6.

25. Penney SE, Bruce IA, Saeed SR. Botulinum toxin is effective and safe for palatal tremor: a report of five cases and a review of the literature. J Neurol 2006;253:857–60.

26. Park SN, Bae SC, Lee GH, et al. Clinical characteristics and therapeutic response of objective tinnitus due to middle ear myoclonus: a large case series. Laryngoscope 2013;123:2516–20.

27. Dong C, Zhao PF, Yang JG, et al. Incidence of vascular anomalies and variants associated with unilateral venous pulsatile tinnitus in 242 patients based on dual-phase contrast-enhanced computed tomography. Chin Med J 2015;128:581–5.

28. Harvey RS, Hertzano R, Kelman SE, et al. Pulse-synchronous tinnitus and sigmoid sinus wall anomalies: descriptive epidemiology and the idiopathic intracranial hypertension patient population. Otol Neurotol 2014;35:7–15.

29. Narvid J, Do HM, Blevins NH, et al. CT angiography as a screening tool for dural arteriovenous fistula in patients with pulsatile tinnitus: feasibility and test characteristics. AJNR Am J Neuroradiol 2011;32:446–53.

Imaging Interpretation of Temporal Bone Studies in a Patient with Tinnitus
A Systematic Approach

Christian L. Stanton, MD, Girish M. Fatterpekar, MD*

KEYWORDS

- Tinnitus • Pulsatile tinnitus • Tinnitus imaging

KEY POINTS

- Tinnitus is a common symptom that is heterogeneous in presentation, pathophysiology, and imaging manifestations.
- Causes are myriad and a multidisciplinary approach is often required.
- Although pulsatile tinnitus is less common, its causes are more readily identified clinically and radiographically.

BACKGROUND (EPIDEMIOLOGY, PATHOPHYSIOLOGY, AND ANATOMY: CLINICAL PERSPECTIVE)

Tinnitus can be broadly defined as an auditory perception of internal origin. It represents a variety of aural sensations, including high or low frequencies that can be constant or intermittent in character. Tinnitus is not a diagnosis but a symptom with a potpourri of possible causes and correspondingly divergent pathophysiologic, anatomic, diagnostic, and therapeutic considerations. Epidemiologic studies have produced disparate chronic tinnitus prevalence estimates mostly in the range of 8% to 20% in the Western world, the variability likely owing to the heterogeneity of tinnitus and inconsistency with respect to methodology. Although it can present at any point in life, its incidence increases with age as well as in the presence of a variety of comorbidities and other symptoms, including hearing loss. It can be a source of persistent angst in a subset of patients and in 20% of tinnitus sufferers the severity is such that their quality of life is significantly impaired.[1-5] This article aims to provide a summary of the imaging findings of structural causes of tinnitus, several of which are discussed in greater depth elsewhere in this issue.

Tinnitus may occur as a result of direct or, more frequently, indirect effects on the auditory system. It can be classified into the pulsatile and nonpulsatile varieties. Pulsatile tinnitus is often the result of nonlaminar flow and among other disease may arise from vascular or neoplastic causes, the latter of which is often based on microvascular shunting. Nonpulsatile tinnitus can result from dysfunction at any point along the ascending auditory system, often as a result of lesions that also cause hearing loss.[6-9]

Within the external auditory canal and middle ear, conditions such as otitis, stapedius or tensor tympani myoclonus, and a variety of middle ear masses may cause tinnitus.[1-3] In the bony labyrinth, conditions such as otosclerosis and Paget disease can be causative, which may be due to mechanical effects or intraosseous arteriovenous shunting.[1,2,10,11] Within the membranous

The authors have no disclosures.
Department of Radiology, NYU Langone Medical Center, 660 1st Avenue, New York, NY 10016, USA
* Corresponding author. Department of Radiology, NYU School of Medicine, New York, NY 10016.
E-mail address: Girish.Fatterpekar@nyumc.org

Neuroimag Clin N Am 26 (2016) 207–225
http://dx.doi.org/10.1016/j.nic.2015.12.009

neuroimaging.theclinics.com

labyrinth, conditions such as Meniere disease or neoplasms such as endolymphatic sac tumors (ELSTs) may directly involve the endolymphatic system.[1,12] A variety of medications may directly affect the cochlear hair cells but can also have more central toxicity in producing tinnitus. Some of the more common causes of pulsatile tinnitus may result from altered cerebrospinal fluid (CSF) pulsations and bone conduction transmitted to the cochlea, as suspected in idiopathic intracranial hypertension (IIH) and several vascular diseases.[13,14] At the level of the internal auditory canal (IAC) and cerebellopontine angle (CPA) cistern, vestibular schwannomas are a frequently implicated culprit.[15–17] Vascular loops may also contact the vestibulocochlear nerve within the IAC or at the level of the cisternal segment and, in some people, elicit tinnitus.[18] Other multifaceted diseases can affect the vestibulocochlear nerve, including Chiari 1 malformations in which inferior brainstem descent may stretch the vestibulocochlear nerve and lead to tinnitus.[19] A variety of intraparenchymal insults such as microangiopathic and demyelinating diseases may cause tinnitus, including those within the hindbrain in which lesions involving the Guillain-Mollaret triangle may manifest indirectly via myoclonus.[1,20] More recently, numerous studies have shown evidence of functional abnormalities within the midbrain, thalamus, and various regions of the cerebral cortex, including the auditory cortex, as being responsible for tinnitus in the absence of findings on conventional imaging.[21–23] Given its prevalence, tinnitus is a frequently encountered condition. Unfortunately, even after extensive work-up, a diagnosis is not discernible in approximately 60% of tinnitus sufferers.[12] This highlights the need to maximize diagnostic yield, which begins by clinical stratification of the patients and often necessitates a multidisciplinary approach. Careful consideration of the explicit character of the tinnitus, attention to precipitating factors, and the presence of concomitant signs and symptoms can help guide the workup. In addition, a neurotologic examination is a must in the workup of tinnitus. Tinnitus is principally categorized as either pulsatile, which can be subjective or objective, or nonpulsatile, which is almost always subjective.[24] When possible, pulsatile tinnitus symptoms should be further subdivided into arterial causes, which are often synchronous with the heartbeat, and venous causes which are sometimes alleviated by compression of the internal jugular vein.[2] For a detailed discussion on the clinical evaluation of tinnitus, (See Hertzano R, Teplitzky TB, Eisenman DJ: Clinical evaluation of tinnitus, in this issue.)

IMAGING APPROACH
Imaging Perspective

Pulsatile tinnitus has a broad range of reported imaging yield with most published estimates in the range of 57% to 100%. Conversely, almost all patients with nonpulsatile tinnitus do not have imaging abnormalities. Further complicating the picture, a diversity of lesions and anatomic variants that can be responsible for either type of tinnitus are also seen in the imaging of other patients in the absence of tinnitus. This last consideration may, in fact, be responsible for the variability in the published imaging yield.[1,2]

There are multitudes of tinnitus imaging algorithms that have been advocated and published but currently there is no broadly accepted expert consensus.[1,2,8,9] There are in fact multiple ways to arrive at a correct diagnosis in the imaging of tinnitus and the various modalities are often complementary, with a general algorithm proposed in **Fig. 1**. Cost and patient safety are important considerations but the manner in which the imaging workup proceeds may frequently be based on institutional preference or availability and thus the authors advocate some general guidelines.

Imaging Guidelines

In nonpulsatile tinnitus, the diagnosis of IAC or CPA cistern masses may be the most significant

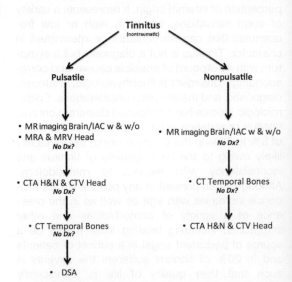

Tinnitus
(nontraumatic)

Pulsatile — Nonpulsatile

- MR imaging Brain/IAC w & w/o
- MRA & MRV Head
  No Dx?

- CTA H&N & CTV Head
  No Dx?

- CT Temporal Bones
  No Dx?

- DSA

- MR imaging Brain/IAC w & w/o
  No Dx?

- CT Temporal Bones
  No Dx?

- CTA H&N & CTV Head

Fig. 1. Suggested approach to the imaging evaluation of the patient with tinnitus. It is reasonable to begin the diagnostic process with CT, then proceed to MR imaging if it is unrevealing, especially in patients with venous pulsatile tinnitus. CT, computed tomography; CTV, CT venogram; DSA, digital subtraction angiography; dX, diagnosis; H&N, head and neck; w, with; w/o, without.

pretest considerations and their presence is best assessed with MR imaging IAC protocol with and without contrast.[3,24] As an example, the authors' institution's protocol is detailed in **Table 1**.

Similarly, most instances of pulsatile tinnitus merit assessment with MR imaging IAC with and without contrast. A typical MR imaging protocol is described in **Table 1**. In addition intracranial MR angiogram (MRA) and MR venogram (MRV) provide significant complementary information and, therefore, are recommended in the imaging work-up. Some institutions suggest use of contemporaneous time-resolved (4-dimensional) MRA sequences allowing for noninvasive dynamic assessment with a temporal resolution in the range of 1 millisecond and elucidation of a variety of vascular diseases not readily discernible on routine imaging.[25] An alternative approach, especially if a suspicion for venous tinnitus and idiopathic intracranial hypertension exists, may be to begin with a CT of the temporal bones and a CT venogram (See Michael A. Reardon MA, Raghavan P: Venous abnormalities leading to tinnitus-imaging evaluation, in this issue). Should these be negative, CT angiogram (CTA) of the head and neck and Doppler carotid sonography are reasonable noninvasive adjuncts to look for causes such as atherosclerotic stenosis, among other causes. Digital subtraction angiography (DSA) can often be reserved as a tertiary modality to fully exclude small vascular malformations. The imaging workup and the radiologist's approach to interpreting imaging studies in patients with tinnitus must, therefore, be guided by an understanding of the clinical scenario. If there is loud, objective pulsatile tinnitus or other strong clinical suspicion

for a vascular malformation, then consideration could be given to DSA as an earlier, more definitive option and to potentially allow for prompt endovascular treatment. In the setting of an abnormal otoscopic examination suggesting a middle ear mass or evidence for osseous disease, a high-resolution temporal bone CT would be the more appropriate first study.[24] In the setting of acute onset of symptoms, particularly with a history of trauma, other severe conditions, such as carotid dissection, should be considered and may be initially worked up by a CTA of the head and neck, which is often readily available.[26] Other imaging studies, such as temporomandibular joint MR imaging, are uncommonly performed but can be used in appropriate clinical scenarios when other studies do not provide any diagnostic information. Knowledge of the clinical situation also helps determine the search pattern while examining these imaging studies. For example, a history of pulse synchronous tinnitus, obliterated by pressure on the internal jugular vein should prompt close scrutiny of the sigmoid sinus wall for dehiscences and diverticula and of the brain and orbits for signs of intracranial hypertension. A history of a reddish mass in the middle ear on otoscopy should guide a search for paragangliomas, jugular bulb abnormalities, and otosclerosis, and warrants close attention to the mesotympanum and hypotympanum, the jugular foramen, and bony labyrinth. It is important to remember that dural arteriovenous fistulae may not be immediately apparent on cross-sectional imaging and subtle signs such as asymmetrically prominent vessels and irregularity of venous sinus walls, for example, must be carefully sought. Some advanced imaging techniques such as functional MR imaging have provided insight in the research of tinnitus and may eventually find a role in the clinical realm.[22] For a discussion on the role of advanced imaging techniques in tinnitus, (See Raghavan P, Steven A, Gandhi D: Advanced neuroimaging of tinnitus, in this issue.)

DIFFERENTIAL DIAGNOSIS

An exhaustive discussion of the myriad causes that can cause tinnitus is impractical. This article, therefore, focuses on some of the more common causes and a few unusual but important causes responsible for tinnitus. Given the realities of imaging yield (see previous discussion), the focus will inherently trend toward diseases more frequently associated with pulsatile tinnitus but we will also highlight some causes more typically associated with nonpulsatile tinnitus.

Table 1
MR imaging brain or IAC protocol example

Precontrast	Postcontrast (half-dose, weight-based)
Trace-ADC-diffusion whole brain axial 5 mm	T1 fat saturated IAC axial 3 mm
FLAIR Whole Brain Axial 5 mm	T1 IAC coronal 3 mm
[a]CISS IAC 1 mm	[b]Radial VIBE IAC 2 mm
—	T1 whole brain axial 5 mm

Abbreviations: ADC, apparent diffusion coefficient; CISS, constructive interference steady state; VIBE, volumetric interpolated breath-hold examination.
[a] 3D-stimulated T2 gradient-echo siemens sequence.
[b] 3D T1 gradient-echo siemens sequence.

VASCULAR CAUSES
Vascular Malformations

Arteriovenous fistulae (AVF) and arteriovenous malformations (AVMs) are common causes of pulsatile tinnitus. In fact, they are the most common causes in patients with objective pulsatile tinnitus and a normal otoscopic examination.[27]

Arteriovenous fistulae

AVF are characterized by an anomalous direct communication between an artery and vein without interposed vascular nidus. They are thought to be acquired and can be the sequela of trauma, infection, or venous sinus thrombosis. Dural AVF are most frequently supplied by branches of the external carotid artery, and those draining via the transverse and sigmoid sinuses may be the most common ones to cause tinnitus.[2] However, other AVF may be implicated, including those with cortical venous or leptomeningeal drainage, cavernous carotid fistulae, and even those within the scalp, face, and neck.[1,10,24] MR imaging findings in AVF can include prominent flow voids, with associated intracranial hemorrhage and/or intraparenchymal hyperintensity (ie, edema, infarction, or gliosis).

Arteriovenous malformations

AVMs are usually pial-based lesions characterized by an abnormal connection between artery and vein with interposed vascular nidus. There are several subtypes based on differences in angioarchitecture and location, any of which may present as tinnitus.[1,24] They are generally thought to be congenital; however, they most frequently present in the third or fourth decades of life. Intracranial AVMs are usually supplied by branches of the internal carotid arteries or the vertebrobasilar system. MR imaging findings in intra-axial AVM include a tangle of flow voids (so-called bag of worms) most frequently located in the cerebral hemispheres. AVMs carry an approximately 4% annual risk of hemorrhage but a variety of characteristics may alter their course.[28] While evaluating the imaging features of these lesions, the radiologist should vigilantly assess for the presence of findings that may herald a more aggressive clinical course, such as flow-related or intranidal aneurysms, and a pattern of diffuse leptomeningeal vein prominence, the so-called pseudophlebitic pattern.[29]

MRA using dynamic sequences will show arteriovenous shunting as early filling veins in most of these vascular malformations and can provide critical details about lesion character and complexity for classification and treatment planning, most closely rivaling the diagnostic capabilities of DSA.[30] Despite the utility of these modern MRA techniques, DSA remains the gold standard in the setting of vascular malformations and allows for endovascular treatment when appropriate (**Fig. 2**).

Acquired Arterial Diseases

Aneurysms

Aneurysms can occasionally present as pulsatile tinnitus, most notably those arising from the

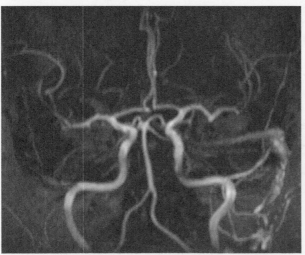
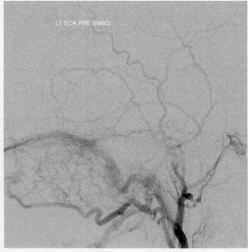

Fig. 2. Dural arteriovenous fistula. Maximum intensity projection time-of-flight MR angiogram (MRA) (*left*) depicts flow-related enhancement within the carotid and vertebrobasilar intracranial arterial system, as well as abnormal prominent enhancement of left external carotid artery branches, and left transverse and sigmoid sinuses. Selective left external carotid artery injection DSA (*right*) confirms presence of a dural arteriovenous fistula supplied by an enlarged left occipital artery with multiple small vessels communicating with the left transverse and sigmoid sinuses.

petrous carotid artery. It is theorized that this may be in part due to compressive obliteration of the adjacent venous plexus that may normally act to dampen the carotid pulsations. With the loss of this buffer, the pulsations within the aneurysm may then be transmitted either directly or via a bone conduction mechanism to the cochlea.[31] However, other mechanisms can contribute. For example, in the setting of aneurysm rupture, hemorrhage itself can result in acute tinnitus as 1 of several symptoms.[32] On an MR imaging study, a petrous carotid aneurysm can be confused with a variety of petrous apex mass lesions. However,

a CTA should provide unequivocal evidence for the correct diagnosis (Fig. 3).

Arterial dissection

Arterial dissection can be seen in multiple settings, including trauma, and may occasionally produce pulsatile tinnitus, particularly when involving the extracranial internal carotid arteries. When present, additional symptoms of cerebral ischemia or Horner syndrome will typically coexist with tinnitus. If clinically suspected, angiographic evaluation should be promptly undertaken via CTA, DSA, or MRA to facilitate treatment initiation. The

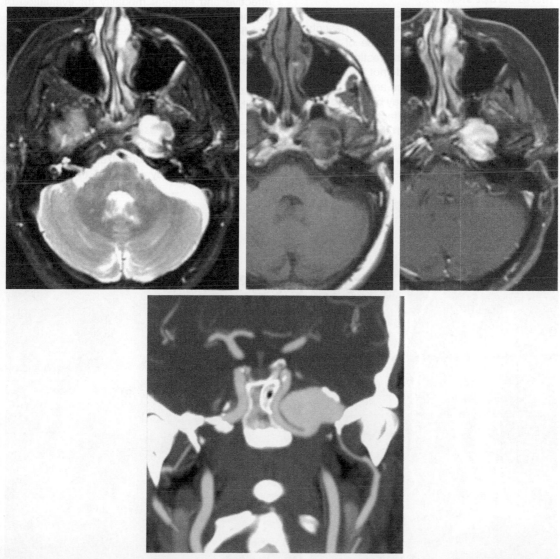

Fig. 3. Petrous internal carotid artery aneurysm. Top: Axial T2 weighted (T2W) (*right*), precontrast T1 weighted (T1W) (*middle*), and postcontrast T1W (*left*) images depict a T2 hyperintense, T1 hypointense enhancing expansile lesion centered at the left petrous apex. Bottom: Coronal CTA image confirms a large saccular aneurysm arising from the horizontal petrous segment of the left internal carotid artery. (*Courtesy of* S. Sabat, MD, University of Alabama at Birmingham.)

most frequent finding on both CTA and time-of-flight MRA is smooth, tapered (flame-shaped) narrowing of the vessel lumen. When available, an MRA may be the best modality and should also include a fat suppressed axial T1 weighted (T1W) sequence through the neck (**Fig. 4**) as well as a diffusion-weighted sequence of the brain. The former allows evaluation for a potentially compressive intramural thrombus or hematoma that will appear as a hyperintense crescent, whereas the latter allows evaluation for presence of ischemic infarcts, which is an important factor when considering anticoagulation.[24]

Atherosclerotic stenosis

Atherosclerotic stenosis, particularly involving the extracranial carotid arteries, has been described as the second-most frequent cause of pulsatile tinnitus in at least 1 study.[2,33] Interestingly, the laterality and degree of stenosis do not always correlate with the tinnitus symptoms and the cause of the tinnitus in these patients may be a direct result of turbulent flow, an indirect effect of sympathetic activation or some combination thereof. However, atherosclerotic carotid stenosis treated with endarterectomy has been shown to relieve tinnitus symptoms in some patients.[2] Subclavian steal

phenomenon is most frequently due to atherosclerotic stenosis at the subclavian artery origin and can also present with tinnitus. The mechanism of tinnitus in this setting is purportedly related to anastomoses between the vertebral artery and the occipital artery.[2] CTA has several advantages compared with DSA, MRA, and ultrasound in these settings. Specifically, CTA offers high spatial resolution, allows for accurate discrimination of atherosclerotic plaque composition (ie, soft or calcific), and fosters elucidation of coexistent diseases such as ulceration and dissection. However, Doppler carotid sonography avoids exposure to ionizing radiation and may also be the most cost-effective and efficient modality for evaluation of the neck vessels.[34] Ultrasound can depict turbulent flow via spectral broadening while accurately grading most stenoses via peak systolic velocity measurement. In suspected subclavian steal, both sonography and MRA can reliably show flow reversal in the vertebral artery, which is not feasible by conventional CTA.

Fibromuscular dysplasia

Fibromuscular dysplasia is an idiopathic angiopathy that affects medium-sized arteries and is seen most frequently in young to middle-aged

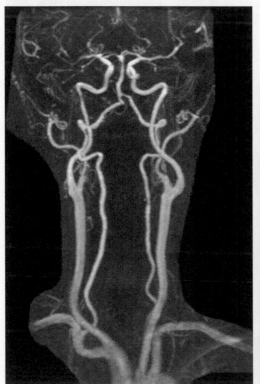
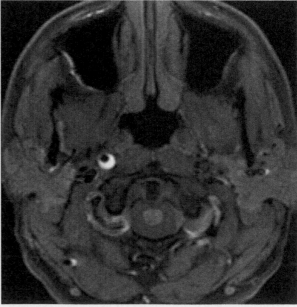

Fig. 4. Internal carotid artery dissection. Left: Contrast-enhanced MRA depicts mild focal narrowing at the distal cervical segment of the right internal carotid artery. Right: The dissection is best depicted on this axial T1W fat saturation image, with an intramural hematoma seen as a hyperintense crescent.

women. Cerebrovascular involvement, particularly of the carotid arteries, is not infrequent in this condition, being second only to the renal arteries. With carotid involvement, tinnitus is the second-most common presenting symptom after cerebral ischemic symptoms and is seen in approximately 30% of patients.[12] As with carotid stenosis, the mechanism of the symptoms may be some combination of several factors and may be further exacerbated by the frequent coexistence of renovascular hypertension in these patients. Whether seen on carotid sonography or any angiographic study, the classic pathognomonic appearance of fibromuscular dysplasia is the string-of-beads sign, reflecting the segmental corrugated morphology of the vessels (**Fig. 5**). However, it may also present with stenosis, typically high in the cervical segment internal carotid artery. Potential cerebrovascular sequelae for which the radiologist must remain alert include aneurysms (seen in 30% of cases), spontaneous dissections (seen in 10%–20%), and focal ischemic infarcts.[10] Thus, brain MR imaging and intracranial MRA are also highly recommended in these patients.

Congenital Arterial Variants

Aberrant internal carotid artery
An aberrant internal carotid artery is an anatomic variant seen in approximately 1% of the

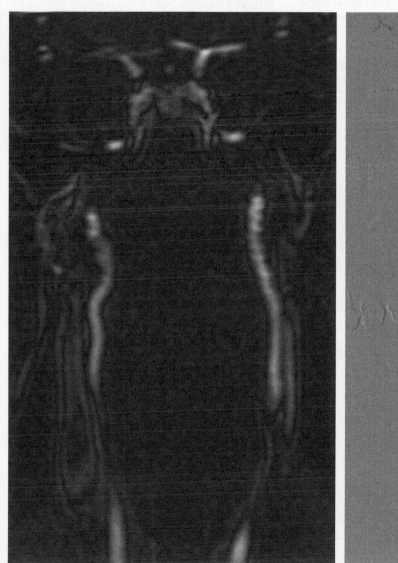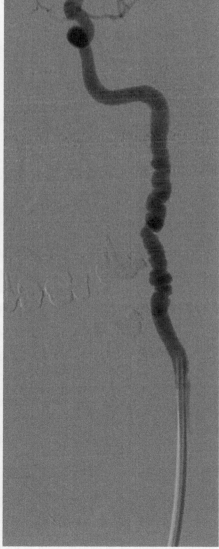

Fig. 5. Fibromuscular dysplasia. Segmental corrugated string-of-beads appearance of bilateral cervical internal carotid arteries on neck time-of-flight MRA (*left*). In a different patient, DSA study demonstrates a string-of-beads appearance of the left cervical internal carotid artery (*right*).

population, most of whom are asymptomatic.[35] However, a subset of these people present with symptoms including pulsatile tinnitus and conductive hearing loss. This variant represents agenesis of the normal cervical segment internal carotid artery with corresponding persistence and enlargement of the inferior tympanic artery, normally an embryologic branch of the ascending pharyngeal artery. This artery travels into the middle ear via the inferior tympanic canaliculus (also known as Jacobson canal), where it may be seen otoscopically as a red anterior middle ear mass. The artery then anastomoses with an enlarged caroticotympanic artery and finally continues as the horizontal segment of the petrous carotid artery.

Unfortunately, the portion of this vessel within the middle ear along the cochlear promontory can be mistaken for a soft tissue mass such as a glomus tympanicum on otoscopic examination.[10] However, the constellation of imaging findings should clearly delineate these entities and prompt the radiologist to offer no differential diagnosis for this normal variant. On temporal bone CT, these findings include the tubular appearance of the middle ear density, enlargement of the inferior tympanic canaliculus and atresia of the carotid canal (Fig. 6). On MRA or other angiographic studies a characteristic "7" configuration will be seen in the coronal projection, resulting from the abnormally lateral course of the artery into the middle ear and the unique angulation as it turns toward the petrous carotid. Focal wall dehiscence is more frequently seen in the aberrant internal carotid artery variant than the normal internal carotid

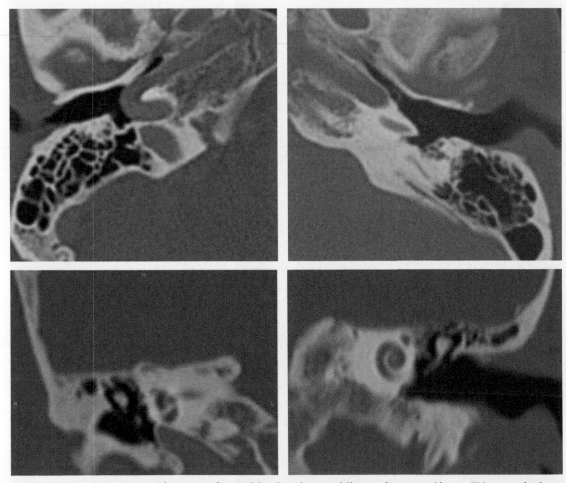

Fig. 6. Aberrant internal carotid artery. Left: Axial (*top*) and coronal (*bottom*) temporal bone CT images depict an abnormal lateral course of the right aberrant internal carotid artery as it traverses the middle ear via the enlarged inferior tympanic canaliculus anterior to the jugular bulb. There is dehiscence at its lateral apex as it loops around the cochlear promontory. Subsequently, it continues anteromedially and narrows before it connects to the horizontal petrous segment of the internal carotid artery. Right: Axial (*top*) and coronal (*bottom*) temporal bone CT scans depict the normal appearance of the left internal carotid artery for reference.

artery and the radiologist should be attentive to this possibility.

Persistent stapedial artery

A persistent stapedial artery (PSA) is extremely rare but, when present, it can frequently coexist with the more common aberrant internal carotid artery.[36] As with the aberrant internal carotid, whereas most people with this variant are asymptomatic, pulsatile tinnitus and conductive hearing loss can occur. The stapedial artery is normally a transient embryologic vessel that functions as an anastomosis between the external and internal carotid arteries. When it persists, it extends from the carotid canal and courses through the middle ear along the cochlear promontory and via the obturator foramen of the stapes. It then courses along the tympanic and geniculate portions of the facial nerve and exits the middle ear cavity to supply blood to the territory typically supplied by the middle meningeal artery. The PSA may be too small to be appreciated by MRA. However, on temporal bone CT a linear soft tissue density may be seen, giving the appearance of a pseudo duplicated facial nerve canal in the coronal plane and a Y-shaped enlargement of the geniculate fossa in the axial plane. A secondary finding that can be an important clue to the attentive radiologist is atresia or absence of the foramen spinosum, which is due to arrested development of the middle meningeal artery (**Fig. 7**).

Venous Causes

In recent years, there has been greater recognition of previously under-reported causes of tinnitus localizable to the venous system. The character of tinnitus in such causes can differ considerably from that of arterial causes and sometimes presents as a venous hum. These forms of tinnitus can sometimes be modulated by the application of direct compression on the ipsilateral jugular vein. Restraint must be exercised in making a definitive diagnosis in patients with such findings, however, because they are often present in individuals without tinnitus symptoms.[2]

Sigmoid sinus diverticula and dehiscence

Sigmoid sinus diverticula and dehiscence is one of the findings that has recently gained traction as an underdiagnosed cause of tinnitus and has been described as the most common venous cause by some investigators.[30] In sigmoid sinus diverticula, there is protrusion of the dural sinus into the mastoid portion of the temporal bone. The primary theory is that pulsatile tinnitus is elicited by nonlaminar flow in this outpouching and then transmitted via bone conduction to the cochlea.[31] An association with IIH has been described and it

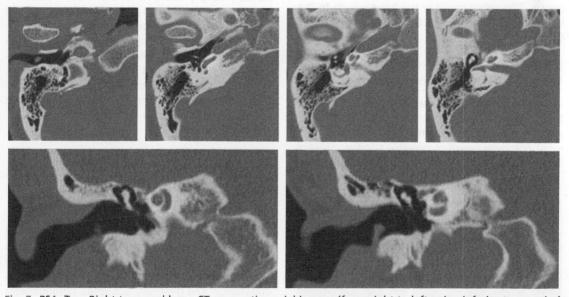

Fig. 7. PSA. Top: Right temporal bone CT consecutive axial images (from *right to left* going inferior to superior) demonstrate a tubular soft density representing a PSA arising from the lateral aspect of the carotid canal (*far right*), faintly seen traversing superiorly and anteriorly within the middle ear along the cochlear promontory (*middle left and middle right*) and parallel to the tympanic segment of the facial nerve (*far left*). Absence of the foramen spinosum is also depicted. Bottom: Right temporal bone CT consecutive coronal images depict a pseudo duplicated facial nerve canal appearance resulting from the presence of PSA at the inferior margin of the cochlear promontory.

has also been postulated that sigmoid sinus diverticula may be a manifestation of intracranial hypertension on a spectrum with dural venous sinus stenosis[30] (see later discussion). The imaging findings of sigmoid sinus diverticula and dehiscence are best depicted on temporal bone CT. Although development of dehiscence offers a plausible explanation for why often the tinnitus onset may be sudden in such patients, this finding may be overestimated by imaging,[30] highlighting the need for caution when interpreting this entity. For a comprehensive overview of sigmoid sinus wall anomalies and their surgical management (See Michael A. Reardon MA, Raghavan P: Venous abnormalities leading to tinnitus-imaging evaluation, in this issue.)

High-riding jugular bulb
High-riding jugular bulb is usually considered to be present when the superior margin of the jugular bulb extends above the floor of the IAC. This finding has reported incidence ranges between 4% and 20%. Among those patients, about 5% have pulsatile tinnitus.[2] The likely mechanism for tinnitus may be via bone conduction of nonlaminar venous flow to the closely apposed cochlea. Jugular bulb dehiscence can also cause tinnitus and may coexist with a high-riding jugular bulb or be seen as a separate entity (Fig. 8). In such cases, the clinician may be able to deduce its presence by visualizing a bluish hypotympanic mass on otoscopy. The relationship of the jugular bulb to the IAC is usually best depicted on temporal bone CT coronal images.[3]

INTRACRANIAL PRESSURE ABNORMALITIES
Idiopathic Intracranial Hypertension

IIH is characterized by elevated CSF pressure in the absence of a mass lesion or other discernable cause. It is considered by many to be the most common cause of pulsatile tinnitus, present in 40% of patients in some series.[1,37] Headaches

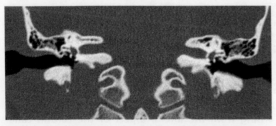

Fig. 8. Dehiscent jugular bulb. High-resolution CT temporal bone coronal scan demonstrates a markedly thinned or dehiscent right jugular bulb. However, the right jugular bulb is not high riding. A normal left jugular bulb is seen.

are the most common symptom in IIH patients but pulsatile tinnitus is present in about 60% and is most frequently unilateral.[38] As its name suggests, the pathogenesis of IIH remains elusive; however, it is strongly correlated with obesity and the female gender and has been attributed to underabsorption of CSF.[39] Additionally, an association with dural venous sinus stenosis, particularly of the transverse sinus, is well described but somewhat controversial and has been reciprocally proposed as both a sequela of IIH as well as a possible cause.[14,40] A popular proposed mechanism of pulsatile tinnitus in IIH patients suggests that the elevated intracranial pressures facilitate transmission of arterial pulsation through the CSF, which in turn compresses the dural venous sinus walls and converts flow from laminar to nonlaminar within the sinuses.[37] There is also a strong association between IIH and sigmoid sinus wall anomalies (See Michael A, Reardon MA, Raghavan P: Venous abnormalities leading to tinnitus-imaging evaluation, in this issue). The nature of this association, however, remains to be clarified. Although imaging for IIH is insensitive, there are some signs that are quite useful when present; especially flattening of the optic discs, reported as only 44% sensitive but 100% specific (Fig. 9). Other findings sometimes associated with IIH include dilation and tortuosity of the optic nerve sheaths, an enlarged or partially empty sella, and slit-like ventricles.[41] However, given the relative insensitivity of MR imaging, invasive CSF pressure measurement remains the gold standard when evaluating IIH. A possible complication is permanent visual deficits, therefore prompt treatment initiation is important.[40] The first line of treatment in most patients is weight loss and diuretics but, in some patients, more invasive measures such as CSF shunting are required.

Intracranial Hypotension

Intracranial hypotension presents in patients primarily as orthostatic headaches but other symptoms, including tinnitus, can coexist.[12,40] The source of the low intracranial pressure is often a CSF leak and, although the most common cause is idiopathic (ie, spontaneously from a dural defect), a preceding lumbar puncture is not uncommon.[40] The generally accepted pathogenesis relates to the Monroe-Kellie doctrine, which dictates that the intracranial volume remains constant and thus any reduction in CSF must be compensated by increase in another component. The typical first manifestation of this is an increase in intracranial blood volume but, in more severe

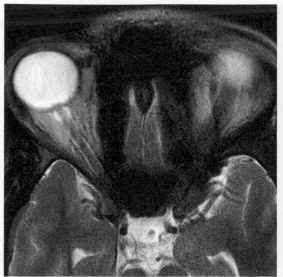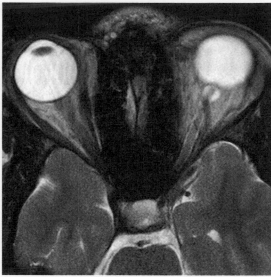

Fig. 9. IIH. Axial T2W MR imaging depict flattening of bilateral optic discs and prominent optic nerve sheath complexes. A partially empty sella turcica is also suggested.

cases, subdural fluid collections can accumulate, possibly secondary to increased microvascular permeability and fluid transudation.[40] The shift in intracranial volume explains some of the characteristic imaging features including diffuse pachymeningeal enhancement on contrast-enhanced MR imaging (in about 83%), pituitary hyperemia, and subdural collections (in about 17%). The frequent presence of brain sagging is thought to be primarily due to dissipated buoyancy from CSF hypovolemia but may be further exacerbated in the presence of subdural collections. In as many as 43% of cases, the downward brain shift can be severe enough to cause cerebellar tonsillar herniation and can mimic a Chiari 1 malformation.[40] The resultant traction on the vestibulocochlear nerve is a potential shared mechanism of tinnitus with Chiari 1 patients; however, in intracranial hypotension, it may alternatively result from abnormal pressure transmission to the cochlear perilymph.[42] If conservative management (ie, bed rest and caffeine) does not persistently alleviate the symptoms, intracranial hypotension often responds favorably to spinal epidural blood patch.

NEOPLASMS

Most neoplasms that cause tinnitus are benign, which may simply reflect the predominance of such lesions in the temporal bone region. The most common causes of nonpulsatile tinnitus with a radiologic correlate are CPA cistern or IAC masses but these may also occasionally cause pulsatile tinnitus.[2,24] Conversely, the most common middle ear masses typically present with pulsatile tinnitus and may be subjective or objective.[27]

Posterior Fossa Masses

Vestibular schwannomas

Vestibular schwannomas are the most common posterior fossa tumor in adults, representing 80% to 90% of masses in this region and constituting up to 10% of intracranial neoplasms overall.[15] Histopathologically these represent benign neoplasms arising from the glial-Schwann cell junction along the vestibulocochlear nerves, most frequently involving the superior vestibular nerve within the IAC at the level of the porus acusticus. The symptoms from vestibular schwannomas frequently include slowly progressive and asymmetric sensorineural hearing loss but unilateral tinnitus can be present in up to 80% and may be the isolated presenting symptom in about 10% of individuals.[16,17] These symptoms can result from direct compression of the vestibulocochlear nerve or from compression of its blood supply.[1] Almost all are unilateral (about 95%) and they most frequently present in the fifth or sixth decade of life. Bilaterality and earlier presentation are hallmarks of neurofibromatosis type 2, an autosomal dominant condition also characterized by presence of meningiomas and ependymomas.

Variable but typically slow growth on the order of a couple millimeters per year can yield expansion of the porus acusticus as well as extension into the CPA cistern. There are overlapping imaging features with other posterior fossa masses that can cause tinnitus such as CPA cistern meningiomas with IAC extension. However, some findings are more characteristic of schwannomas, including acute angles relative to the skull base, heterogeneous enhancement, and IAC expansion (Fig. 10). Radiologic assessment must describe mass extent and regional anatomy to assist potential surgical or radiosurgical planning. This includes consideration of positions of the venous structures to help the surgeon decide on the feasibility of translabyrinthine versus suboccipital or middle cranial fossa approaches. Unfortunately, although surgical or radiosurgical interventions may prevent progression of the neoplasm and related symptoms, tinnitus is inconsistently ameliorated by these efforts suggesting permanent damage to the nerve.[3]

Endolymphatic sac tumors

ELSTs are rare, slow-growing, but invasive, tumors situated at the retrolabyrinthine posterior fossa. They typically present in the second or third decades of life with sensorineural hearing loss and tinnitus in up to 92%.[43] Histopathologically they arise from the endothelium of the endolymphatic sac and are usually classified as papillary cystadenomas.[44] ELSTs are seen in approximately 16% of patients with Von-Hippel Lindau syndrome and they are bilateral in 30% of these patients. Possible mechanisms for both hearing loss and tinnitus include direct invasion of the temporal bone or endolymphatic hemorrhage and hydrops.[12,43] On CT, typical findings include permeative changes at the petrous temporal bone and intratumoral calcifications sometimes described as bony sequestra or spicules

(Fig. 11). On MR imaging, findings are variable but they may enhance and can have heterogeneous intrinsic T1 and T2 signal intensity that may reflect some combination of intralesional hemorrhage and vascular flow voids.[44]

Jugular Fossa and Middle Ear Masses

Paragangliomas

Paragangliomas are benign, hypervascular neuroendocrine tumors with several subtypes. These are found most frequently in women in the fifth and sixth decades of life.[45] Histopathologically, these masses arise from neural crest progenitor cells that differentiate into chemoreceptors (glomus cells) and are intimately associated with both blood vessels and nerves. Paragangliomas presenting with tinnitus usually arise within the jugular foramen or middle ear.

A paraganglioma isolated to the jugular fossa represents a glomus jugulare. Avid enhancement and close apposition to the jugular vein as well as occasional heterogeneous signal intensity within the vein can make it difficult to assess for jugular vein invasion on MR imaging; therefore, MRV can be particularly useful in this setting. Several imaging features can distinguish glomus jugulare from other jugular foramen masses such as schwannomas. CT demonstrates permeative osseous changes. MR demonstrates a classic salt-and-pepper appearance on noncontrast T1W image; salt representing hemorrhage and pepper suggestive of flow voids. Following contrast administration, typically intense enhancement is seen. These tumors can grow laterally into the tympanic cavity, sometimes via an (enlarged)

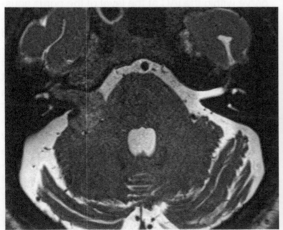
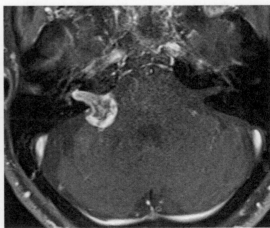

Fig. 10. Vestibular schwannoma. High-resolution constructive interference steady state (CISS) axial MR imaging through the IAC (*left*) depict an intermediate signal intensity mass, expanding the IAC and extending laterally into the CPA cistern where it causes mass effect on the right middle cerebellar peduncle. Postcontrast T1W axial MR imaging through the IAC (*right*) depicts heterogeneous enhancement of the mass.

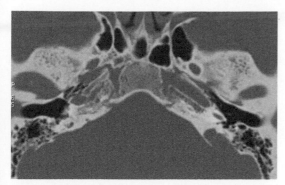

Fig. 11. ELST. Axial temporal bone CT image depicts a destructive lesion involving the left temporal bone at the retrolabyrinthine petrous portion in the expected location of the vestibular aqueduct. Faint hyperdense spicules are seen within the lesion suggestive of ELST.

inferior tympanic canaliculus and are then known as glomus jugulotympanicum (**Fig. 12**). Glomus jugulotympanicum can also reflect several paragangliomas occurring along Jacobson nerve or sometimes Arnold nerve.[1,2,10]

An isolated, circumscribed soft tissue middle ear mass typically along the cochlear promontory with an intact hypotympanic floor represents the glomus tympanicum. The glomus tympanicum usually arises along the inferior tympanic branch of the glossopharyngeal nerve, the other name for Jacobson nerve. This nerve travels in the inferior tympanic canaliculus, usually alongside the inferior tympanic artery before traversing the medial aspect of the middle ear. It is the most common tumor of the middle ear and often the diagnosis of a glomus tumor at this site can be suggested clinically with the combination of pulsatile tinnitus and a red retrotympanic mass on otoscopy.[2,24] However, imaging is still warranted to definitively differentiate from other causes, such as an aberrant internal carotid artery, as well as to characterize lesion extent. A well-defined rounded soft tissue mass on the cochlear promontory is highly suggestive of glomus tympanicum. Contrast administration is not always necessary to make the diagnosis. If contrast is

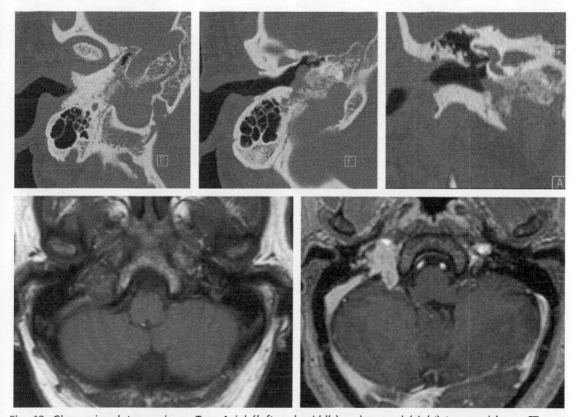

Fig. 12. Glomus jugulotympanicum. Top: Axial (*left* and *middle*) and coronal (*right*) temporal bone CT scans depict a soft tissue mass along the cochlear promontory of the middle ear with permeative changes at the petrous temporal bone and expansion of the jugular fossa. Bottom: Precontrast T1W axial image (*left*) depicts a mass involving the right mesotympanum and jugular fossa with heterogeneous-salt and-pepper signal intensity. Postcontrast T1W axial image (*right*) confirms presence of an enhancing mass extending between these compartments likely via the inferior tympanic canaliculus.

administered, like glomus tumors at other sites, intense enhancement is seen.

Facial nerve schwannomas

Facial nerve schwannomas can occur anywhere along the course of the facial nerve resulting in a variety of possible presentations that include conductive or sensorineural hearing loss and tinnitus in addition to facial palsy. These lesions are relatively rare compared with schwannomas involving other nerves, particularly the common vestibular variety. On otoscopy, those involving the middle ear may appear as a fleshy white retrotympanic mass. As with their presentation, the imaging appearance of these schwannomas is variable but can include a lobulated or tubular homogeneously enhancing soft tissue mass.[46] Depending on the involved facial nerve segment there may also be smooth expansion of the surrounding bone (Fig. 13). The possible mechanism of tinnitus produced by facial nerve schwannomas is not completely understood.[47]

Facial nerve hemangiomas

Facial nerve hemangiomas are rare, benign facial nerve lesions with potential for similar presentation as facial nerve schwannomas, including tinnitus. Hemangioma, in this case, is a misnomer because these are in fact venous vascular malformations that involve the venous plexus around the facial

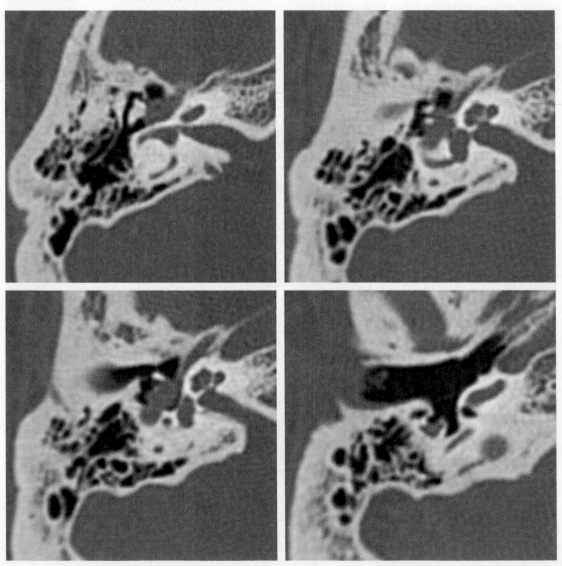

Fig. 13. Facial nerve schwannoma. Consecutive axial temporal bone CT images depict a lobulated soft tissue mass involving the anterior genu, tympanic, posterior genu and mastoid segments of the right facial nerve with associated expansion of the facial nerve canal.

nerve. Typically, these are slow-growing lesions found most frequently at the geniculate fossa where they tend to also produce facial nerve paralysis and, occasionally, at the fundus of the IAC where they can also cause sensorineural hearing loss.[3] The typical imaging appearance on CT is a honeycomb configuration with indistinct margins as a result of marginal osseous permeation and superimposed hyperdense stippling, all of which can help distinguish from schwannomas. On MR imaging, they are most frequently hyperintense on both T1 and T2 and avid enhancement may be seen in a heterogeneous or homogeneous pattern[3,12] (Fig. 14). For a detailed discussion on Paragangliomas, vascular skull base tumors and their endovascular management (See Woolen S, Gemmete JJ: Paragangliomas of the head and neck, in this issue.)

OSSEOUS CAUSES
Otosclerosis

Otosclerosis (also known as otospongiosis) is an osseous dysplasia that is characterized by bone resorption and remodeling, which results in replacement of the normal enchondral temporal bone with hypervascular haversian bone. Although still considered idiopathic, it is likely that genetic and immunologic components are contributory because this condition is seen almost exclusively in whites, and has a predominance in middle-aged women.[48] A frequent clinical presentation is with various forms of hearing loss and, contrary to some earlier accounts, tinnitus may be encountered in most of these patients, in the range of 65% to 91%,[1,49] and can even precede hearing loss.

There are 2 distinct forms of otosclerosis. The more common fenestral subtype represents about 85% of cases and is characterized by involvement of the fissula ante fenestram, a fibrocartilaginous

cleft located anterior to the oval window. This subtype more typically produces conductive hearing loss but can progress to involve the otic capsule, in which case it can yield a mixed pattern. The retrofenestral subtype is characterized by involvement of the bone around the basal turn of the cochlea, is typically associated with sensorineural hearing loss, and may more frequently have coexistent vestibular symptoms. Temporal bone CT best depicts the findings in otosclerosis, with characteristic areas of demineralization in the early phase and sclerosis in the later phase (Figs. 15 and 16). In the early phase, this may include a low attenuation ring around the intrinsically circumscribed cochlea, resulting in a so-called double-ring sign. In the late phase, findings may include heaped-up sclerotic margins near the oval window.[1] MR imaging is generally insensitive for otosclerosis but may depict T2 hyperintensity or pericochlear enhancement in the early phase.[1,3]

The tinnitus in otosclerosis is most frequently nonpulsatile in nature but can be pulsatile in a minority of cases, likely reflecting different pathophysiology. Bony deposition around the stapes can result in stapedial ankylosis, which has been implicated as the mechanical cause of hearing loss as well as tinnitus in many of these patients.[11] Stapedectomy with placement of a stapes prosthesis can successfully treat hearing loss as well as tinnitus in a significant proportion of them, particularly those with nonpulsatile forms. The minority of otosclerosis patients with pulsatile tinnitus, however, may have an alternative primary contributing component, namely the vascular proliferation of the haversian bone with associated arteriovenous shunting.[1,10,12,37] On otoscopy, resultant hyperemic mucosa can occasionally be visualized as a pink blush near the cochlear promontory, the so-called Schwartz sign.[2,24]

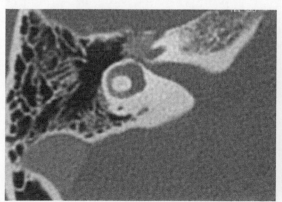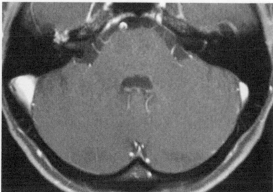

Fig. 14. Facial nerve hemangioma. Axial temporal bone CT image (*left*) depicts the typical honeycomb appearance of a facial nerve hemangioma centered at the right geniculate ganglion. Postcontrast T1W axial image (*right*) depicts avid enhancement of the hemangioma.

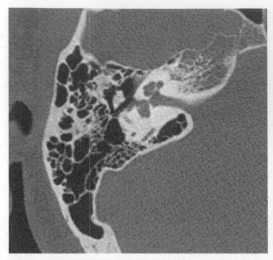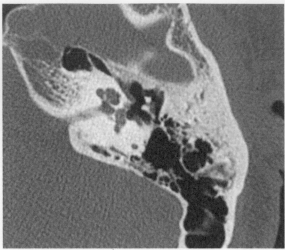

Fig. 15. Fenestral otosclerosis. Subtle focal demineralization is depicted at the fissula ante fenestra, just anterior to the left oval window consistent with fenestral otosclerosis (*right*). The normal right side is shown for comparison (*left*).

Paget Disease

Paget disease is another osseous disorder that can involve the skull in 25% to 65% of patients, of whom a significant proportion may have tinnitus as a symptom.[50] As with otosclerosis, it remains an idiopathic condition but may have genetic and inflammatory components. It affects approximately 3% of the population over the age of 40 and usually affects whites and men.[10] Paget has 3 characteristic histopathologic phases of variable osseous resorption and deposition that are reflected grossly in the varying distributions of bony changes. The mechanism of pulsatile tinnitus in these patients seems to be related to the associated intraosseous vascular proliferation and arteriovenous shunting, as also

suggested with some forms of otosclerosis.[1,10,12] Temporal bone CT is again the preferred radiologic modality for depicting this osseous abnormality. Unlike otosclerosis, the distribution of Paget is more diffuse throughout the skull base and sometimes produces a classic cotton-wool appearance (**Fig. 17**). A paucity of maxillofacial involvement, as well as the older age of presentation, are key features in differentiating Paget from fibrous dysplasia.

MISCELLANEOUS CAUSES
Meniere Disease

Meniere disease is characterized by intermittent symptoms of vertigo, sensorineural hearing loss, tinnitus, and aural fullness. This clinical diagnosis

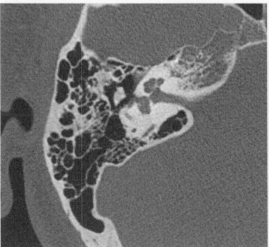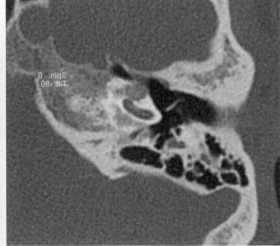

Fig. 16. Retrofenestral otosclerosis. Confluent areas as well as patchy areas of demineralization are shown within the left temporal bone with a predominance around the basal turn of the cochlea (*right*). The normal right side is shown for comparison (*left*).

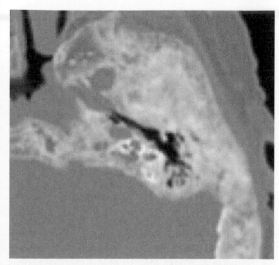

Fig. 17. Paget disease. Diffuse heterogeneous bone mineralization with a cotton-wool appearance and expansion of the diploic space involving the visualized left temporal bone suggestive of Paget disease.

is thought to be the result of endolymphatic hydrops with multiple possible causes, including trauma, infection, and inflammatory processes. At a population level, subtle imaging changes of the membranous labyrinth and semicircular canals in particular have been described. However, routine assessment and detection of such subtle findings has not been clinically applicable, thus imaging has historically played a limited role in Meniere. Novel imaging methods may change this in the near future. One such recently

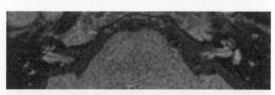

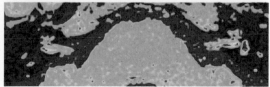

Fig. 18. Meniere disease. High-resolution postcontrast FLAIR CISS image (*top*) with double gadolinium dose on 3T depicts diminished enhancement in the right labyrinthine structures in a patient with right-sided nonpulsatile tinnitus. The fused color maps provide increased imaging sensitivity for Meniere disease (*bottom*). (*From* Hagiwara M, Roland JT Jr, Wu X, et al. Identification of endolymphatic hydrops in Ménière's disease utilizing delayed postcontrast 3D FLAIR and fused 3D FLAIR and CISS color maps. Otol Neurotol 2014;35(10):e340; with permission.)

described technique uses high-resolution postcontrast fluid-attenuated inversion recovery (FLAIR) constructive interference steady state (CISS) imaging and double gadolinium dose on 3T MR imaging with a specificity of 97%[51] (**Fig. 18**). In about one-third of patients, the symptoms of Meniere resolve spontaneously, although a variety of possible treatments, including surgery and medication injections, have shown variable benefits with response in about half of patients.

SUMMARY

Tinnitus is a tricky symptom that is complex to evaluate. A myriad of causes exist. The workup, therefore, is extensive. The radiologist plays a key role in the evaluation of tinnitus. Knowing the type of tinnitus (ie, pulsatile or nonpulsatile variant) can help appropriately set a protocol to better evaluate these cases. Although imaging evaluation typically remains focused to the temporal bone, assessing the rest of the intracranial structures and head and neck may be necessary for a thorough assessment.

REFERENCES

1. Vattoth S, Shah R, Cure JK. A compartment-based approach for the imaging evaluation of tinnitus. AJNR Am J Neuroradiol 2010;31:211–8.
2. Kang M, Escott E. Imaging of tinnitus. Otolaryngol Clin North Am 2008;41:179–93.
3. Branstetter BF, Weissman JL. The radiologic evaluation of tinnitus. Eur Radiol 2006;16:2792–802.
4. Axelsson A, Ringdahl A. Tinnitus—a study of its prevalence and characteristics. Br J Audiol 1989; 23(1):53–62.
5. Landgrebe M, Azevedo A, Baguley D, et al. Methodological aspects of clinical trials in tinnitus: a proposal for an international standard. J Psychosom Res 2012;73:112–21.
6. Møller AR. Pathophysiology of tinnitus. In: Sismanis A, editor. Otolaryngol clin north Am. Amsterdam: WB Saunders; 2003. p. 249–66.
7. Waldvogel D, Mattle HP, Sturzenegger M, et al. Pulsatile tinnitus: a review of 84 patients. J Neurol 1998;245(3):137–42.
8. Sismanis A. Pulsatile tinnitus. In: Hughes GB, Pensak ML, editors. Otolaryngol clin north Am. New York: Thieme; 2003. p. 445–60.
9. Crummer RW, Hassan GA. Diagnostic approach to tinnitus. Am Fam Physician 2004;69:120–6.
10. Moonis G, Lo WM, Maya MM. Vascular tinnitus of the temporal bone. In: Som PM, Curtin HD, editors. Head and neck imaging. 5th edition. St Louis (MO): Mosby; 2011. p. 1409–25.

11. Stankovic KM, McKenna MJ. Current research in otosclerosis. Curr Opin Otolaryngol Head Neck Surg 2006;14:347–51.

12. Marsot-Dupuch K. Pulsatile and nonpulsatile tinnitus: a systemic approach. Semin Ultrasound CT MR 2001;22:250–70.

13. Sohmer H, Freeman S. Further evidence for a fluid pathway during bone conduction auditory stimulation. Hear Res 2004;193:105–10.

14. Farb RI, Vanek I, Scott JN, et al. Idiopathic intracranial hypertension: the prevalence and morphology of sinovenous stenosis. Neurology 2003;60:1418–24.

15. Cummings CW, Arriaga M, Brackmann D, et al. Otolaryngology–head and neck surgery. 5th edition. Philadephia: Elsevier; 2005. p. 3803–40.

16. Moffat DA, Baguley DM, Beynon GJ, et al. Clinical acumen and vestibular schwannoma. Am J Otol 1998;19:82–7.

17. Baguley DM, Humphriss RL, Axon PR, et al. The clinical characteristics of tinnitus in patients with vestibular schwannoma. Skull Base 2006;16(2):49–58.

18. De Ridder D, De Ridder L, Nowé V, et al. Pulsatile tinnitus and the intrameatal vascular loop: why do we not hear our carotids? Neurosurgery 2005;576: 1213–7.

19. Wiggs WJ Jr, Sismanis A, Laine FJ. Pulsatile tinnitus associated with congenital central nervous system malformations. Am J Otol 1996;17:241–4.

20. Oliveira CA, Negreiros J Jr, Cavalcante IC, et al. Palatal and middle-ear myoclonus: a cause for objective tinnitus. Int Tinnitus J 2003;9(1):37–41.

21. Mühlau M, Rauschecker JP, Oestreicher E, et al. Structural brain changes in tinnitus. Cereb Cortex 2006;16:1283–8.

22. Lanting CP, De KE, Bartels H, et al. Functional imaging of unilateral tinnitus using fMRI. Acta Otolaryngol 2008;128(4):415–21.

23. Llinas R, Urbano FJ, Leznik E, et al. Rhythmic and dysrhythmic thalamocortical dynamics: GABA systems and the edge effect. Trends Neurosci 2005; 28(6):325–33.

24. Weissman JL, Hirsch BE. Imaging of tinnitus: a review. Radiology 2000;216(2):342–9.

25. Zou Z, Ma L, Cheng L, et al. Time-resolved contrast-enhanced MR angiography of intracranial lesions. J Magn Reson Imaging 2008;27:692–9.

26. Narvid J, Do HM, Blevins NH, et al. CT angiography as a screening tool for dural arteriovenous fistula in patients with pulsatile tinnitus: feasibility and test characteristics. AJNR Am J Neuroradiol 2011;32: 446–53.

27. Remley KB, Coit WE, Harnsberger HR, et al. Pulsatile tinnitus and the vascular tympanic membrane: CT, MR, and angiographic findings. Radiology 1990;174:383–9.

28. Kim EJ, Vermeulen S, Li FJ, et al. A review of cerebral arteriovenous malformations and treatment

with stereotactic radiosurgery. Transl Cancer Res 2014;3(4):399–410.

29. Willinsky R, Goyal M, Brugge K, et al. Tortuous, engorged pial veins in intracranial dural arteriovenous fistulas: correlations with presentation, location, and MR findings in 122 patients. AJNR Am J Neuroradiol 1999;20:1031–6.

30. Grewal AK, Kim HY, Comstock RH, et al. Clinical presentation and imaging findings in patients with pulsatile tinnitus and sigmoid sinus diverticulum/ dehiscence. Otol Neurotol 2014;35(1):16–21.

31. De Ridder D. Pulsatile tinnitus. In: Møller AR, Langguth B, De Ridder D, et al, editors. Textbook of tinnitus. New York: Springer; 2011. p. 467–75.

32. Moonis G, Hwang CJ, Ahmed T, et al. Otologic manifestations of petrous carotid aneurysms. AJNR Am J Neuroradiol 2005;26(6):1324–7.

33. Sismanis A, Stamm MA, Sobel M. Objective tinnitus in patients with atherosclerotic carotid artery disease. Am J Otol 1994;15(3):404–7.

34. Titi M, George C, Bhattacharya D, et al. Comparison of carotid Doppler ultrasound and computerised tomographic angiography in the evaluation of carotid artery stenosis. Surgeon 2007;5(3): 132–6.

35. Botma M, Kell RA, Bhattacharya J, et al. Aberrant internal carotid artery in the middle-ear space. J Laryngol Otol 2000;114:784–7.

36. Silbergleit R, Quint DJ, Mehta BA, et al. The persistent stapedial artery. AJNR Am J Neuroradiol 2000; 21:572–7.

37. Sismanis A. Pulsatile tinnitus: a 15-year experience. Am J Otol 1998;19:472–7.

38. Shaw GY, Millon SK. Benign intracranial hypertension: a diagnostic dilemma. Case Rep Otolaryngol 2012;2012:814696.

39. Boulton M, Armstrong D, Flessner M, et al. Raised intracranial pressure increases CSF drainage through arachnoid villi and extracranial lymphatics. Am J Physiol 1998;275(3):889–96.

40. Yuh EL, Dillon WP. Intracranial hypotension and intracranial hypertension. Neuroimaging Clin N Am 2010;20:597–617.

41. Agid R, Farb RI, Willinsky RA, et al. Idiopathic intracranial hypertension: the validity of cross-sectional neuroimaging signs. Neuroradiology 2006;48(8): 521–7.

42. Portier F, Monteguiaga C, Rey E, et al. Spontaneous intracranial Hypotension: A rare cause of labyrinthine hydrops. Ann Otol Rhinol Laryngol 2002;112: 817–20.

43. Lonser RR, Kim HJ, Butman JA, et al. Tumors of the endolymphatic sac in von Hippel–Lindau disease. N Engl J Med 2004;350:2481–6.

44. Friedman RA, Hoa M, Brackmann DE. Surgical management of endolymphatic sac tumors. J Neurol Surg 2013;74(01):012–9.

45. Hoeffner EG, Mukherji SK, Ghandhi D, et al, editors. Temporal bone imaging. New York: Thieme; 2008.

46. Wiggins RH 3rd, Harnsberger HR, Salzman KL, et al. The many faces of facial nerve schwannoma. AJNR Am J Neuroradiol 2006;27:694–9.

47. Kirazli T, Oner K, Bilgen C, et al. Facial nerve neuroma: clinical, diagnostic, and surgical features. Skull Base 2004;14:115–20.

48. Markou K, Goudakos J. An overview of the etiology of otosclerosis. Eur Arch Otorhinolaryngol 2009; 266(1):25–35.

49. Sobrinho PG, Oliveira CA, Venosa AR. Long-term follow-up of tinnitus in patients with otosclerosis after stapes surgery. Int Tinnitus J 2004;10(2):197–201.

50. Mackenzie I, Young C, Fraser WD. Tinnitus and Paget's disease of bone. J Laryngol Otol 2006;120: 899–902.

51. Hagiwara M, Roland JT Jr, Wu X, et al. Identification of endolymphatic hydrops in Ménière's disease utilizing delayed postcontrast 3D FLAIR and fused 3D FLAIR and CISS color maps. Otol Neurotol 2014;35(10):e337–42.

Arterial Abnormalities Leading to Tinnitus

Timothy R. Miller, MD[a],*, Yafell Serulle, MD, PhD[a], Dheeraj Gandhi, MBBS, MD[a,b]

KEYWORDS

- Tinnitus • Pulsatile tinnitus • Vascular abnormalities • Internal carotid artery variants
- Vascular masses

KEY POINTS

- Tinnitus is the unwanted perception of sound in the absence of an external stimulus, and is classified by whether the sound is perceived by the patient alone, or also by the clinician (eg, subjective vs objective), and by whether it is continuous, or varies with the patient's pulse (eg, nonpulsatile vs pulsatile).
- Causes of pulsatile tinnitus can broadly be divided into vascular and nonvascular types.
- Vascular causes of pulsatile tinnitus are numerous, and are further characterized by the location of the source of the noise within the cerebral-cervical vasculature: arterial, arteriovenous, and venous.
- Patients with pulsatile tinnitus should first be evaluated with contrast-enhanced CT of the head and temporal bones. When noninvasive imaging studies fail to demonstrate a cause, catheter angiography should be performed to exclude a dural arteriovenous fistula.

INTRODUCTION

Tinnitus is the unwanted perception of sound that originates, or seems to originate, from one or both ears.[1–4] The word tinnitus is derived from the Latin *tinnire*, meaning "to ring," although the noise may also be described as buzzing, roaring, whistling, clicking, or musical.[5–8] Chronic, persistent tinnitus may affect up to 10% of adults in the general population, although only a minority of these cases are severe.[4,6,9–11] Tinnitus occurs more frequently in men than women, and increases in prevalence with advancing age, being most common from 40 to 70 years.[2–6,11] However, tinnitus has also been reported in children.[3–6,11,12] The perceived severity of tinnitus may have little correlation with its impact on the patient's life, which may range from negligible to disabling.[3,5–9]

Tinnitus may be classified by whether the sound is perceived by the patient alone, or also by the clinician (eg, subjective vs objective), and by whether it is continuous, or varies with the patient's pulse (eg, nonpulsatile vs pulsatile).[1,2,4–6,8,13] Most cases of tinnitus are subjective and nonpulsatile, with the auditory stimulus being present without an external stimulus.[1,3,8,9,11] In these instances, tinnitus is often associated with some degree of hearing loss and is thought to likely arise from damage to the outer hair cells of the inner ear.[1,3] Imaging typically is unremarkable in these cases.[5] Treatment options for this type of tinnitus primarily consist of patient reassurance, masking devices, and cognitive therapy.[3,11,12] However, nonpulsatile tinnitus can rarely be associated with a treatable condition, such as a tumor compressing the eighth

---

Disclosure Statement: The authors have nothing to disclose.
[a] Division of Interventional Neuroradiology, Department of Diagnostic Radiology, University of Maryland School of Medicine, 22 South Green Street, Baltimore, MD 21201, USA; [b] Departments of Radiology, Neurology and Neurosurgery, University of Maryland School of Medicine, 22 South Green Street, Baltimore, MD 21201, USA
* Corresponding author.
E-mail address: tmiller5@umm.edu

cranial nerve or other central nervous system processes, including stroke or demyelinating disease.[5]

In contradistinction, pulsatile tinnitus, where the perceived sound is synchronous with the patient's pulse, is relatively uncommon, accounting for less than 10% of tinnitus cases.[1,6,10,14] Pulsatile tinnitus is often secondary to an identifiable, acquired vascular anomaly or congenital vascular variant, which produces a physical sound that is perceived by the inner ear, and may sometimes be auscultated by the clinician.[4,5,7,8,10,11,14–16] Because the source of the sound is often unilateral, pulsatile tinnitus also typically localizes to one side.[1] However, cases of bilateral pulsatile tinnitus do occur, but are more likely to be nonvascular in origin, and are typically associated with sensorineural hearing loss.[1,17] Imaging plays an important role in the management of pulsatile tinnitus by helping to evaluate for potential causes, which can then facilitate treatment.[1,7,8,18]

PATHOPHYSIOLOGY OF VASCULAR PULSATILE TINNITUS

Pulsatile tinnitus resulting from a vascular cause may be generated by two possible pathophysiologic mechanisms. First, turbulent blood flow at the skull base near the inner ear may generate the noise, which in turn can be generated by a focal vascular stenosis and/or increased blood flow.[1,2,5,6,14,19] Alternatively, pulsatile tinnitus may be generated by amplification of normal blood flow sounds at the skull base.[1] This can occur because of changes in the inner ear that result either in increased bone conduction of sound, or abnormal sound conduction leading to a loss of normal masking of external noise.[1] However, the exact etiologic relationship between these mechanisms and the production of tinnitus needs to be established.[5]

ETIOLOGIES OF PULSATILE TINNITUS

Numerous causes of pulsatile tinnitus have been described in the literature, the frequency of which have varied considerably between individual reports.[1,6,10] This likely reflects differences in diagnostic work-up and patient selection among the various studies.[1,10] However, the most commonly identified causes of pulsatile tinnitus include benign intracranial hypertension, atherosclerotic disease with associated arterial stenosis, vascular anatomic variants, and vascular tumors at the skull base.[1,3,10,13,19–21] In general, a cause of pulsatile tinnitus is identified in up to 70% of cases.[1,7] An underlying cause of pulsatile tinnitus is more likely to be found when the symptom is unilateral

compared with bilateral, and when the tinnitus is objective.[1,10]

Causes of pulsatile tinnitus can broadly be divided into vascular and nonvascular types.[6] Nonvascular causes include palatal, tensor tympani, and stapedial myoclonus; a patulous Eustachian tube; certain drugs; dehiscent semicircular canal; and chronic middle ear disease.[4,6,10,15,17] Vascular etiologies of pulsatile tinnitus are numerous, and are further characterized by the location of the source of the noise within the cerebral-cervical vasculature: arterial, arteriovenous, and venous.[6] This article focuses on arterial and arteriovenous causes of pulsatile tinnitus. For Venous causes, see Reardon M, Raghavan P: Venous Abnormalities Leading to Tinnitus: Imaging Evaluation, in this issue.

ARTERIAL CAUSES OF PULSATILE TINNITUS
Arteriosclerotic Disease

Arteriosclerotic plaque is one of the most common causes of arterial narrowing in the head and neck, and should be considered in elderly patients presenting with pulsatile tinnitus, particularly in those individuals with a history of hypertension, diabetes, hyperlipidemia, or smoking.[1,6,13,14,17,21] The tinnitus may be generated from turbulent blood flow at the site of arterial narrowing, or conversely from compensatory increased blood flow in a cervical artery secondary to arteriosclerotic occlusion of another vessel.[1,6,13,14,17,21] Tinnitus may occur because of arteriosclerotic plaque arising from any segment of the internal carotid artery (ICA), from the carotid bifurcation to the intracranial carotid siphon, and from plaque involving the subclavian and vertebral-basilar arteries.[5,14] Treatment of the associated arterial stenosis may result in resolution of the tinnitus.[5]

Fibromuscular Dysplasia

Pulsatile tinnitus may also be caused by fibromuscular dysplasia (FMD), a segmental, nonatheromatous vascuolopathy affecting medium-size arteries, which typically presents in young to middle-age women.[1,5,7,10,22–25] FMD most commonly involves the renal and cervical ICAs, although the cervical vertebral arteries may also be affected.[17,22,23] These vessels often display a characteristic beaded appearance, with multifocal areas of vessel irregularity and narrowing, separated by segments of variable dilatation (Fig. 1).[4,17,22,23] Pulsatile tinnitus is presumably generated by turbulent blood flow arising from the associated arterial stenoses and dilatation.[5,22,23] Many cases of FMD are asymptomatic, although patients may experience pulsatile tinnitus, headache, vertigo, transient ischemic attack, and cerebral infarct.[4,5,22,23] Overall, patients

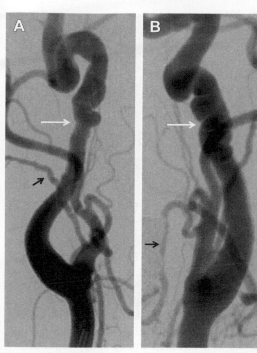

Fig. 1. Bilateral fibromuscular dysplasia. Digital subtraction angiography images illustrate a beaded appearance of the bilateral cervical internal carotid arteries (*white arrows, A* and *B*) in a patient with severe fibromuscular dysplasia. Note also the involvement of several external carotid artery branches (*black arrows, A* and *B*).

with FMD have an excellent prognosis. Asymptomatic patients with involvement of the carotid or vertebral arteries should be placed on antiplatelet therapy (typically 81 mg aspirin), whereas those with symptoms may be treated more aggressively with angioplasty, stenting, or anticoagulation.[26]

Arterial Dissection

Cranial-cervical arterial dissections may cause pulsatile tinnitus in a minority of cases (**Fig. 2**).[1,4,5,7,10,13,17,27] A dissection consists of a tear in the intima of an artery, which allows blood to dissect into the vessel wall. Dissections may be traumatic or spontaneous, and commonly involve the cervical ICAs and distal intracranial vertebral arteries. A significant minority of patients presenting with cervical arterial dissection may have an underlying connective tissue disorder that predisposes to intimal tearing.[28] Acute dissections may produce pulsatile tinnitus by generating turbulent blood flow, either secondary to vessel narrowing from the mural hematoma, or from the formation of a dissecting pseudoaneurysm.[1,4,5,17] Associated signs and symptoms include neck and facial pain, stroke, Horner syndrome, and subarachnoid hemorrhage when the dissection is intracranial.[13,17]

Treatment of cervical arterial dissections is focused on preventing artery-to-artery embolism secondary to thrombus formation at the site of injury. This may be accomplished by placing the patient on either anticoagulation or antiplatelet therapy, depending on the preference of the clinician.[28] Although there are no data in the literature to support the use of anticoagulation over antiplatelet agents, anticoagulation may be preferred when there is an associated hemodynamically significant stenosis or intraluminal thrombus noted on imaging.[28–30] Finally, patients with progressive, hemodynamically significant arterial stenosis associated with the dissection may be offered endovascular stenting to maintain patency of the vessel (see **Fig. 2**).[31–33]

Aberrant Internal Carotid Artery

Anatomic variants involving arteries at the skull base are another potential source of pulsatile tinnitus, the most common of which is the aberrant ICA (**Fig. 3**).[7,14,16,34] Here, the ICA appears to deviate from its normal anteromedial course through the petrous carotid canal to extend laterally into the middle ear.[5,35] This variant is thought to arise when the cervical portion of the ICA fails to develop normally, or regresses.[4,8,10,35] Consequently, two embryonic vessels, the inferior tympanic and caroticotympanic arteries, enlarge to reconstitute the ICA at the level of the missing segment.[4,7,8,10,35] Because the inferior tympanic artery normally extends laterally through the temporal bone and into the medial middle ear via the inferior tympanic canaliculus, the aberrant ICA follows a similar course.[5,10,35] On otologic examination, an aberrant ICA, which may be dehiscent, can appear as a vascular, pulsatile structure located behind the tympanic membrane.[4,5,7,8,34,35] This variant must be noted on imaging to avoid inadvertent biopsy, because these lesions can be mistaken for a glomus tympanicum, with catastrophic consequences.[5,10,34,35]

Isolated Stapedial Artery

Occasionally, an isolated persistent stapedial artery may be a cause of pulsatile tinnitus.[7,8] This vessel is identified as a small artery arising from the petrous ICA, which courses into the hypotypanum and through the obturator foramen, located between the crura of the stapes (**Fig. 4**).[8,10,14] In these instances, the persistent stapedial artery supplies the normal vascular territory of the middle meningeal artery, with the more proximal portion of the middle meningeal artery, and the foramen spinosum, being absent.[5,8,10] A persistent stapedial artery is another potential cause of a vascular retrotympanic mass.[10]

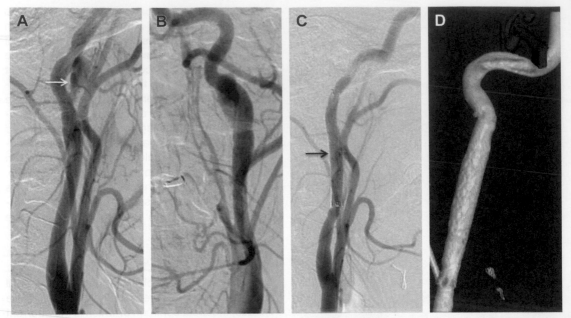

Fig. 2. Middle-age woman who presented with left-sided pulsatile tinnitus and found to have subcranial dissecting aneurysm on CT angiography. Anterior (*A*) and lateral (*B*) digital subtraction angiography images demonstrate a dissection of the left cervical internal carotid artery. Note a large pseudoaneurysm at the distal aspect of the dissected cervical internal carotid artery (*arrow*). Lateral view of a digital subtraction angiography (*C*) and shaded surface display volume-rendered image (*D*) following placement of a covered stent (*arrow*) across the dissection. Note the complete resolution of the pseudoaneurysm. The patient reported complete resolution of the tinnitus following the stent placement.

Dehiscence of the Internal Carotid Artery

Dehiscence of the ICA canal is another anatomic variant that may produce pulsatile tinnitus and present as a vascular retrotympanic mass.[4,10,14] On imaging, thinning or absence of the normal bony covering of the ICA is noted, typically near the basal turn of the cochlea.[4,5] This allows for direct transmission of arterial pulsations to the membranous labyrinth, resulting in pulsatile tinnitus.[14]

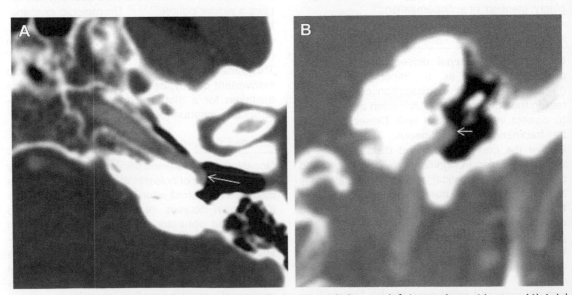

Fig. 3. A 57-year-old woman with history of pulsatile tinnitus and aberrant left internal carotid artery. (*A*) Axial and (*B*) coronal CT angiogram images through the middle ear demonstrate the looping aberrant internal carotid artery (*arrow*) on the cochlear promontory.

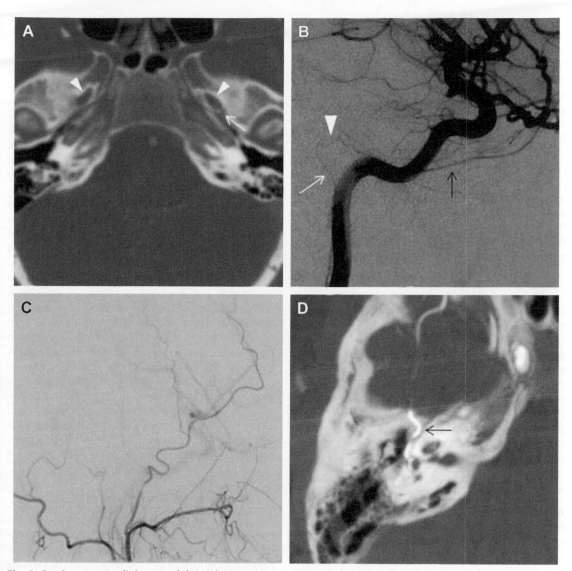

Fig. 4. Persistent stapedial artery. (*A*) Axial CT angiogram image in bone window at the level of the skull base in the area of the foramen ovale (*arrowheads*) reveals absence of the foramen spinosum on the right, with a visible foramen spinosum on the left (*arrow*). (*B*) Lateral right internal carotid artery angiogram demonstrates the persistent stapedial artery (*white arrow*), which arises from the cervical internal carotid artery transitioning into the anterior tympanic segment of the facial nerve canal (*arrowhead*) to supply the middle meningeal artery (*black arrow*). (*C*) Lateral right external carotid angiogram demonstrates absence of the middle meningeal artery branches. (*D*) Axial image from a dynamic CT angiogram demonstrates the stapedial artery along the tympanic part of the facial canal (*arrow*).

Although a dehiscent carotid canal is seen when the vessel takes a normal course through the skull base, an aberrant ICA may also demonstrate this feature as it extends into the middle ear.[4,5]

Arterial Compression of the Vestibulochoclear Nerve

Arterial compression of the eighth cranial nerve has been suggested as a cause of pulsatile tinnitus.[4,10,36,37] Loops of the anterior inferior cerebellar artery often lie in close approximation to the nerve at the cerebellopontine angle and internal auditory meatus, and may generate tinnitus by transmission of arterial pulsations.[5,36] A similar mechanism has been proposed in certain cases of trigeminal neuralgia, with vascular compression of the fifth cranial nerve.[5,37] However, there remains some uncertainty as to whether this mechanism actually plays a role in generating pulsatile tinnitus.[4] First, loops of the anterior inferior cerebellar artery (AICA) are commonly noted to be adjacent to the nerve in asymptomatic patients undergoing high-resolution MRI (up to 14%–34% of the normal population).[1,37] Furthermore, although some authors have noted a significant difference in the frequency of contact between AICA loops and the eighth cranial nerve in symptomatic patients compared with control subjects, others have failed to do so.[10,37–41] However, more recently Nowe and colleagues[42] found an 80-fold higher association of vascular loops in the internal auditory canal in patients with pulsatile tinnitus compared with those with continuous tinnitus on high-resolution T2-weighted MRI. Consequently, this mechanism should be considered when other causes of pulsatile tinnitus have been excluded.

Cerebral Aneurysms

Cerebral aneurysms arising from the internal carotid and vertebral-basilar arteries are a rare cause of pulsatile tinnitus.[1,8,17,43,44] These lesions may produce pulsatile tinnitus by causing turbulent flow in the parent artery.[1] Alternatively, an aneurysm compressing the vestibulocochlear nerve may allow transmission of arterial pulsations.[5] However, despite previously published reports, pulsatile tinnitus remains an uncommon manifestation of aneurysms involving the cerebral-cervical vasculature.[1,44]

Increased Cardiac Output

Any disorder leading to increased cardiac output may produce pulsatile tinnitus. Common causes include anemia, thyrotoxicosis, and pregnancy[3,6,13,14,17] (Box 1).

Box 1
Arterial causes of pulsatile tinnitus

- Vascular stenosis or occlusion
  - Arteriosclerosis
  - Fibromuscular dysplasia
  - Arterial dissection
- Normal variants at the skull base
  - Aberrant internal carotid artery
  - Persistent stapedial artery
  - Dehiscent internal carotid artery
- Arterial compression of the eighth cranial nerve
- Cerebral aneurysms

CAUSES OF PULSATILE TINNITUS ARISING AT THE ARTERIOVENOUS JUNCTION
Paragangliomas

Vascular skull base tumors are another potential cause of pulsatile tinnitus, of which the paraganglioma is the most common.[1,4,7,10,16,17] These lesions are a type of slow-growing neuroendocrine neoplasm that arise from chromaffin-negative glomus cells derived from the embryonic neural crest.[7,10] Most paragangliomas are benign (approximately 97%), but they can be locally destructive with erosion of adjacent bony structures.[7,10] In the head and neck, common locations for these lesions include the middle ear along the cochlear promontory, jugular foramen, and carotid body (glomus jugular, tympanicum, and carotid body tumor respectively).[1,4,7,8,10]

The glomus tympanicum is thought to arise in the middle ear from the tympanic or Jacobson nerve, a branch of the ninth cranial nerve, and can present as a vascular retrotympanic mass.[4,7,8] On computed tomography (CT), a glomus tympanicum typically appears as a rounded soft tissue mass in the middle ear situated along the cochlear promontory, whereas larger paragangliomas (typically glomus jugular or jugulotympanicum) often demonstrate erosion of adjacent osseous structures.[4,7,8,10] On MRI, paragangliomas avidly enhance after gadolinium contrast administration, and large lesions typically exhibit a characteristic, heterogeneous "salt and pepper" appearance.[4,7,8,10]

Other Vascular Skull Base Neoplasms

Additional skull base lesions that have been associated with pulsatile tinnitus include endolymphatic sac tumors, vestibular schawannomas, hemangiopericytomas, meningiomas, cavernous hemangiomas of the middle ear, facial nerve hemangiomas, and vascular metastases to the skull base.[1,4,7,8,10] Endolymphatic sac tumors are aggressive vascular neoplasms arising from the endolymphatic sac, and often present with mixed conductive and sensorineural hearing loss, facial nerve paralysis, and occasionally, pulsatile tinnitus.[10] There is a strong association with von Hippel-Lindau disease.[10] Hemangiopericytomas are an uncommon, aggressive, vascular neoplasms arising from capillary wall pericytes, which may present in the central nervous system as locally invasive, enhancing meningeal masses.[10] Cavernous hemangiomas are rare, benign tumors of the middle ear that may mimic a glomus tympanicum on imaging.[5] Finally, facial nerve hemangiomas typically arise in the region of the geniculate ganglion or internal auditory canal, and may demonstrate calcification on CT.[5] These lesions commonly result in facial nerve paralysis or sensorineural hearing loss depending on their location, but they have also been associated with pulsatile tinnitus.[5]

Vascular Malformations

Dural arteriovenous fistulae (DAVF) arising in the region of the transverse and sigmoid sinuses are a well-known cause of pulsatile tinnitus.[16,17,45–47] DAVF represent roughly 10% of intracranial vascular malformations, and are thought to be acquired lesions secondary to venous thrombosis with subsequent recanalization.[45,46] They are characterized by small arteriovenous shunts arising in the dura matter, typically involving meningeal arteries arising from the external carotid and vertebral arteries.[45,46] Although DAVF can produce intolerable pulsatile tinnitus in some patients, the main risk of these lesions is hemorrhagic stroke and nonhemorrhagic neurologic deficits, which can occur when the fistula recruits cortical veins extending over the surface of the brain.[1,17,45,46] Tinnitus caused by DAVF is objective or subjective, depending on the size of the lesion and the degree of associated arteriovenous shunting. Finally, other vascular malformations of the head and skull base may lead to pulsatile tinnitus, including direct carotid cavernous fistula and arteriovenous malformations.[4,7,8]

Osseous Dysplasias

Osseous dysplasias involving the temporal bone have been associated with pulsatile tinnitus, presumably caused by increased bone vascularity.[5] Otosclerosis is an idiopathic, infiltrative disorder of the petrous temporal bone that results in replacement of portions of the normally dense bony labyrinth by vascular, haversian bone, which can appear radiolucent on CT in the active phase of the disease.[4,5,8,10,14] Although otosclerosis typically results in mixed hearing loss and continuous tinnitus, it has less frequently been associated with pulsatile tinnitus.[4,5,8,10,14,17] Similarly, Paget disease, a nontumorous disorder of bone remodeling that produces disorganized, hypervascular bone, may also cause continuous or pulsatile, and hearing loss, when involving the temporal bone.[4,5,7,10,14,17] Pagetoid bone typically appears expanded and sclerotic on CT, giving a cotton-wool appearance.[4]

Capillary Hyperemia Involving the Temporal Bone

Disorders resulting in capillary hyperemia of the petrous temporal bone are another potential source of pulsatile tinnitus. This includes acute labyrinthitis and microfistulae of the inner ear[1] (Box 2).

VENOUS CAUSES OF PULSATILE TINNITUS

A myriad of disorders involving the venous cerebrocervical vasculature may also result in pulsatile tinnitus. These include intracranial hypertension; acquired stenosis or occlusion of the transverse or sigmoid sinus; dural venous sinus diverticula; and anatomic variants and abnormalities of the skull base and associated veins, including a high-riding jugular bulb, jugular bulb dehiscence, and jugular bulb diverticulum.[1,5,6,48,49] For further information on causes of pulsatile tinnitus, see Woolen S, Gemmete JJ: Paragangliomas of the Head and Neck, in this issue.

DIAGNOSTIC WORK-UP OF TINNITUS

The diagnostic work-up of a patient presenting with tinnitus includes a thorough medical history, physical examination, and targeted laboratory and imaging tests.[1,3,6,17,18] The medical history should note the duration and severity of the tinnitus, factors that make the symptom better or worse, and whether the tinnitus is pulsatile.[1,6] In addition, the patient should be asked about associated otologic symptoms, including hearing loss

---

Box 2
Causes of pulsatile tinnitus arising at the arteriovenous junction

- Vascular skull base tumors
  - Paragangliomas
  - Metastases
  - Meningiomas
  - Cavernous hemangiomas
  - Endolymphatic sac tumors
  - Facial nerve hemangiomas
- Vascular malformations
  - Dural arteriovenous fistulae
  - Direct carotid-cavernous fistula
  - Arteriovenous malformations
- Osseous dysplasias
  - Otosclerosis
  - Paget disease
- Capillary hyperemia
  - Acute labyrinthitis
  - Microfistulae involving the inner ear

and vertigo.[6] Careful attention should be paid to any prior history of trauma to the head and neck, the use of certain medications (eg, angiotensin-converting enzyme inhibitors, calcium channel blockers), diabetes, hypertension, and symptoms suggestive of increased intracranial pressure.[1,6,18] The latter include headache, changes in vision, nausea, and vomiting.[6,17,18]

On examination, careful auscultation of the chest, neck, and skull should be performed to evaluate for heart murmurs, cervical bruits, and objective tinnitus.[3,6,14,15,17] If a bruit is auscultated, certain maneuvers, including carotid artery and internal jugular vein compression, Valsalva, and head rotation, can be performed to evaluate their effect on the bruit, and potentially help determine whether the tinnitus is arterial or venous in etiology.[1,4,10,14,15] A careful otologic examination also needs to be performed to evaluate for a mass or vascular structure behind the tympanic membrane.[3,6,14,17] In addition, blood pressure and body mass index should be measured, and the patient should undergo thorough ophthalmologic and audiologic evaluations.[3,6,8] Finally, laboratory evaluation should include a complete a complete blood count and thyroid function tests, to evaluate for anemia and hyperthyroidism.[3,6,13,17] A lumbar puncture can be performed if there is any clinical suspicion for increased intracranial pressure[1,16] (Box 3).

IMAGING STRATEGIES IN THE EVALUATION OF TINNITUS

Imaging plays an important role in the diagnostic work-up of tinnitus. Cross-sectional studies, such as CT and MRI, are used to evaluate for etiologies of tinnitus in the central nervous system and temporal bone, including benign intracranial hypertension, tumor, otosclerosis, aberrant ICA, and dehiscent semicircular canal.[1,5–7,50] These examinations can then be supplemented by noninvasive vascular imaging to further evaluate for potential vascular causes of tinnitus, including arteriosclerosis or vascular malformations.[2,10] The specific imaging strategy used for an individual patient

---

Box 3
Differential of a vascular retrotympanic mass associated with pulsatile tinnitus

- Glomus tympanicum or jugulotympanicum
- Aberrant or dehiscent internal carotid artery
- Prominent/dehiscent jugular bulb
- Cavernous hemangioma of the middle ear

---

should be tailored to findings on medical history and physical examination, including the quality of the tinnitus (eg, continuous vs pulsatile), results of the otoscopic examination, and whether an objective bruit is present.[4,5,8,51]

In patients presenting with continuous tinnitus and an unremarkable otoscopic examination, MRI of the brain and temporal lobes with contrast is a reasonable first imaging test.[4,5,8,51] In contradistinction, patients with pulsatile tinnitus, or those with a retrotympanic mass on otologic examination, should first be evaluated with contrast-enhanced CT of the head and temporal bones.[4,5,8,51] Finally, if pulsatile tinnitus is associated with an audible bruit on examination, and noninvasive imaging studies fail to demonstrate a cause, catheter angiography should be performed to exclude a DAVF.[8,16,18,51,52]

It is important to remember that imaging findings must be interpreted while considering the patient's overall clinical picture.[1,5] For example, anatomic variants, such as a high-riding jugular bulb or dehiscent internal carotid canal, are often incidentally noted in patients who are either asymptomatic, or whose symptomatology localizes to the contralateral side.[4,5] However, when such a variant is noted ipsilateral to the tinnitus, it may be a plausible explanation for the symptom when other etiologies are excluded. Furthermore, arteriosclerosis is a common finding in older patients, and may be unrelated in an individual presenting with nonpulsatile tinnitus and hearing loss.

NONINVASIVE IMAGING MODALITIES USED IN THE EVALUATION OF TINNITUS

Noninvasive imaging modalities used in the evaluation of pulsatile tinnitus include noncontrast CT, MRI of the head and neck, carotid Doppler ultrasound, and CT and MR angiography and venography. See Raghavan P, Steven A, Gandhi D: Advanced Neuroimaging of Tinnitus, in this issue for detailed information.

INVASIVE IMAGING EVALUATION OF TINNITUS
Catheter Angiography

In cases of objective pulsatile tinnitus where noninvasive imaging fails to disclose a cause, catheter angiography should be performed to exclude a DAVF. Catheter angiography remains the imaging gold standard for DAVF because of its superior temporal and spatial resolution.[45,50] Although CTA or MR angiography may detect larger DAVF by visualizing elements of the fistula (ie, enlarged feeding arteries, small shunts in an affected dural sinus wall), their sensitivity remains low for small lesions.[45,53–56] Alternatively, a catheter angiogram has high sensitivity for detecting DAVF. Furthermore, catheter angiography can fully evaluated all elements of the lesion, including feeding arterial pedicles, site of arteriovenous fistulization, and fistualized draining veins. Catheter angiography may also detect high-risk features of DAVF, including cortical venous drainage, obstruction of draining veins, and venous ectasias.[45,50] Finally, a catheter angiogram is essential for planning of endovascular or surgical treatment when indicated.

Catheter angiography evaluation of pulsatile tinnitus should include selected injections of the bilateral ICAs, external carotid arteries, and vertebral arteries (ie, a six-vessel angiogram). On selection of each vessel, imaging should be performed over the neck and head. On arterial-phase imaging, the selected vessels should be evaluated for stenosis, occlusion, or aneurysm. In addition, the operator must note any variant vessel anatomy, including an aberrant course of the parent vessel; any persistent fetal anatomy (eg, a persistent trigeminal artery); and artery fenestration. The clinician must also pay close attention to the early appearance of draining veins because this may indicate arteriovenous shunting associated with a vascular malformation. Venous-phase imaging should be carefully reviewed for any stenosis, occlusion, or aberrant anatomy involving the dural sinuses and draining veins at the skull base.

SUMMARY

Nonpulsatile tinnitus is a common disorder in the general population, and is frequently associated with injury to the inner ear and sensorineural hearing loss. In contradistinction, pulsatile tinnitus is relatively rare, and often has an underlying structural or vascular cause that may be identified on imaging. The imaging strategy used in a particular case should be tailored to the findings of the patient's medical history and physical examination. If noninvasive imaging fails to demonstrate a cause in a patient with objective pulsatile tinnitus, catheter angiography should be performed to exclude a DAVF.

REFERENCES

1. Hofmann E, Behr R, Neumann-Haefelin T, et al. Pulsatile tinnitus: imaging and differential diagnosis. Dtsch Arztebl Int 2013;110(26):451–8.
2. Krishnan A, Mattox DE, Fountain AJ, et al. CT arteriography and venography in pulsatile tinnitus: preliminary results. AJNR Am J Neuroradiol 2006;27(8):1635–8.
3. Lockwood AH, Salvi RJ, Burkard RF. Tinnitus. N Engl J Med 2002;347(12):904–10.
4. Vattoth S, Shah R, Cure JK. A compartment-based approach for the imaging evaluation of tinnitus. AJNR Am J Neuroradiol 2010;31(2):211–8.
5. Branstetter BF, Weissman JL. The radiologic evaluation of tinnitus. Eur Radiol 2006;16(12):2792–802.
6. Liyanage SH, Singh A, Savundra P, et al. Pulsatile tinnitus. J Laryngol Otol 2006;120(2):93–7.
7. Sonmez G, Basekim CC, Ozturk E, et al. Imaging of pulsatile tinnitus: a review of 74 patients. Clin Imaging 2007;31(2):102–8.
8. Weissman JL, Hirsch BE. Imaging of tinnitus: a review. Radiology 2000;216(2):342–9.
9. Bauer CA. Mechanisms of tinnitus generation. Curr Opin Otolaryngol Head Neck Surg 2004;12(5):413–7.
10. Madani G, Connor SE. Imaging in pulsatile tinnitus. Clin Radiol 2009;64(3):319–28.
11. McFerran DJ, Phillips JS. Tinnitus. J Laryngol Otol 2007;121(3):201–8.
12. Baguley DM, McFerran DJ. Tinnitus in childhood. Int J Pediatr Otorhinolaryngol 1999;49(2):99–105.
13. Sila CA, Furlan AJ, Little JR. Pulsatile tinnitus. Stroke 1987;18(1):252–6.
14. Herraiz C, Aparicio JM. Diagnostic clues in pulsatile tinnitus (somatosounds). Acta Otorrinolaringol Esp 2007;58(9):426–33 [in Spanish].
15. Mattox DE, Hudgins P. Algorithm for evaluation of pulsatile tinnitus. Acta Otolaryngol 2008;128(4):427–31.
16. Remley KB, Coit WE, Harnsberger HR, et al. Pulsatile tinnitus and the vascular tympanic membrane: CT, MR, and angiographic findings. Radiology 1990;174(2):383–9.
17. Sismanis A. Pulsatile tinnitus: contemporary assessment and management. Curr Opin Otolaryngol Head Neck Surg 2011;19(5):348–57.
18. Shin EJ, Lalwani AK, Dowd CF. Role of angiography in the evaluation of patients with pulsatile tinnitus. Laryngoscope 2000;110(11):1916–20.
19. Sismanis A. Pulsatile tinnitus. A 15-year experience. Am J Otol 1998;19(4):472–7.
20. Sismanis A, Smoker WR. Pulsatile tinnitus: recent advances in diagnosis. Laryngoscope 1994;104(6 Pt 1):681–8.
21. Sismanis A, Stamm MA, Sobel M. Objective tinnitus in patients with atherosclerotic carotid artery disease. Am J Otol 1994;15(3):404–7.
22. Dufour JJ, Lavigne F, Plante R, et al. Pulsatile tinnitus and fibromuscular dysplasia of the internal carotid. J Otolaryngol 1985;14(5):293–5.
23. Foyt D, Carfrae MJ, Rapoport R. Fibromuscular dysplasia of the internal carotid artery causing pulsatile tinnitus. Otolaryngol Head Neck Surg 2006;134(4):701–2.
24. Raj RK, Gandhi RT, Katzen BT. Fibromuscular dysplasia-related carotid pseudoaneurysm and pulsatile tinnitus. J Vasc Interv Radiol 2012;23(12):1657.

25. Weihl C, Dorfler A, Forsting M. Pulse synchronous tinnitus as the only symptom of fibromuscular dysplasia of cervical arteries. Rofo 1999;171(4): 334–5 [in German].

26. Olin JW, Pierce M. Contemporary management of fibromuscular dysplasia. Curr Opin Cardiol 2008; 23(6):527–36.

27. Vories A, Liening D. Spontaneous dissection of the internal carotid artery presenting with pulsatile tinnitus. Am J Otolaryngol 1998;19(3):213–5.

28. Debette S, Leys D. Cervical-artery dissections: predisposing factors, diagnosis, and outcome. Lancet Neurol 2009;8(7):668–78.

29. Cervical Artery Dissection in Stroke Study Trial Investigators. Antiplatelet therapy vs. anticoagulation in cervical artery dissection: rationale and design of the Cervical Artery Dissection in Stroke Study (CADISS). Int J Stroke 2007;2(4):292–6.

30. Lyrer P, Engelter S. Antithrombotic drugs for carotid artery dissection. Cochrane Database Syst Rev 2003;(3):CD000255.

31. Cohen JE, Leker RR, Gotkine M, et al. Emergent stenting to treat patients with carotid artery dissection: clinically and radiologically directed therapeutic decision making. Stroke 2003;34(12):e254–7.

32. Kadkhodayan Y, Jeck DT, Moran CJ, et al. Angioplasty and stenting in carotid dissection with or without associated pseudoaneurysm. AJNR Am J Neuroradiol 2005;26(9):2328–35.

33. Malek AM, Higashida RT, Phatouros CC, et al. Endovascular management of extracranial carotid artery dissection achieved using stent angioplasty. AJNR Am J Neuroradiol 2000;21(7):1280–92.

34. Davis WL, Harnsberger HR. MR angiography of an aberrant internal carotid artery. AJNR Am J Neuroradiol 1991;12(6):1225.

35. Lo WW, Solti-Bohman LG, McElveen JT Jr. Aberrant carotid artery: radiologic diagnosis with emphasis on high-resolution computed tomography. Radiographics 1985;5(6):985–93.

36. De Ridder D, De Ridder L, Nowe V, et al. Pulsatile tinnitus and the intrameatal vascular loop: why do we not hear our carotids? Neurosurgery 2005; 57(6):1213–7 [discussion: 1213–7].

37. Chadha NK, Weiner GM. Vascular loops causing otological symptoms: a systematic review and meta-analysis. Clin Otolaryngol 2008;33(1):5–11.

38. Gultekin S, Celik H, Akpek S, et al. Vascular loops at the cerebellopontine angle: is there a correlation with tinnitus? AJNR Am J Neuroradiol 2008;29(9):1746–9.

39. Makins AE, Nikolopoulos TP, Ludman C, et al. Is there a correlation between vascular loops and unilateral auditory symptoms? Laryngoscope 1998; 108(11 Pt 1):1739–42.

40. De Carpentier J, Lynch N, Fisher A, et al. MR imaged neurovascular relationships at the cerebellopontine angle. Clin Otolaryngol Allied Sci 1996;21(4):312–6.

41. McDermott AL, Dutt SN, Irving RM, et al. Anterior inferior cerebellar artery syndrome: fact or fiction. Clin Otolaryngol Allied Sci 2003;28(2):75–80.

42. Nowe V, De Ridder D, Van de Heyning PH, et al. Does the location of a vascular loop in the cerebellopontine angle explain pulsatile and non-pulsatile tinnitus? Eur Radiol 2004;14(12):2282–9.

43. Austin JR, Maceri DR. Anterior communicating artery aneurysm presenting as pulsatile tinnitus. ORL J Otorhinolaryngol Relat Spec 1993;55(1):54–7.

44. Kim DK, Shin YS, Lee JH, et al. Pulsatile tinnitus as the sole manifestation of an internal carotid artery aneurysm successfully treated by coil embolization. Clin Exp Otorhinolaryngol 2012;5(3):170–2.

45. Miller TR, Gandhi D. Intracranial dural arteriovenous fistulae: clinical presentation and management strategies. Stroke 2015;46(7):2017–25.

46. Gandhi D, Chen J, Pearl M, et al. Intracranial dural arteriovenous fistulas: classification, imaging findings, and treatment. AJNR Am J Neuroradiol 2012; 33(6):1007–13.

47. Kusmierska M, Gac P, Nahorecki A, et al. Cranial dural arteriovenous fistula as a rare cause of tinnitus: case report. Pol J Radiol 2013;78(4):65–9.

48. Mehall CJ, Wilner HI, LaRouere MJ. Pulsatile tinnitus associated with a laterally placed sigmoid sinus. AJNR Am J Neuroradiol 1995;16(4 Suppl):905–7.

49. Russell EJ, De Michaelis BJ, Wiet R, et al. Objective pulse-synchronous "essential" tinnitus due to narrowing of the transverse dural venous sinus. Int Tinnitus J 1995;1(2):127–37.

50. Dietz RR, Davis WL, Harnsberger HR, et al. MR imaging and MR angiography in the evaluation of pulsatile tinnitus. AJNR Am J Neuroradiol 1994;15(5):879–89.

51. Willinsky RA. Tinnitus: imaging algorithms. Can Assoc Radiol J 1992;43(2):93–9.

52. Waldvogel D, Mattle HP, Sturzenegger M, et al. Pulsatile tinnitus–a review of 84 patients. J Neurol 1998; 245(3):137–42.

53. Chen JC, Tsuruda JS, Halbach VV. Suspected dural arteriovenous fistula: results with screening MR angiography in seven patients. Radiology 1992; 183(1):265–71.

54. Noguchi K, Melhem ER, Kanazawa T, et al. Intracranial dural arteriovenous fistulas: evaluation with combined 3D time-of-flight MR angiography and MR digital subtraction angiography. AJR Am J Roentgenol 2004;182(1):183–90.

55. Pekkola J, Kangasniemi M. Posterior fossa dural arteriovenous fistulas: diagnosis and follow-up with time-resolved imaging of contrast kinetics (TRICKS) at 1.5T. Acta Radiol 2011;52(4):442–7.

56. Narvid J, Do HM, Blevins NH, et al. CT angiography as a screening tool for dural arteriovenous fistula in patients with pulsatile tinnitus: feasibility and test characteristics. AJNR Am J Neuroradiol 2011; 32(3):446–53.

Venous Abnormalities Leading to Tinnitus
Imaging Evaluation

Michael A. Reardon, MD[a], Prashant Raghavan, MBBS[b],*

KEYWORDS

- Tinnitus • Idiopathic intracranial hypertension • Dehiscent sigmoid sinus
- Sigmoid sinus diverticulum • Dehiscent jugular bulb • Posterior fossa emissary veins

KEY POINTS

- Venous anomalies are the most commonly identified abnormalities in the work-up for pulse synchronous tinnitus.
- Subtle abnormalities such as focal sigmoid sinus wall dehiscence without diverticulum formation can often be overlooked if not incorporated into the standard search pattern for patients with tinnitus.
- Sigmoid sinus wall anomalies are an increasingly recognized cause for pulse synchronous tinnitus. Innovative treatment options including transmastoid sigmoid sinus wall reconstruction have a high rate of success with resolution of symptoms.

INTRODUCTION

Tinnitus can be categorized as subjective or objective and continuous or pulsatile. Pulse synchronous tinnitus (PST) is a repetitive somatosound commonly caused by vascular flow murmurs.[1,2] PST related to vascular flow murmurs can be the result of numerous arterial causes but only a limited set of venous causes. For detailed discussion on Arterial abnormalities leading to tinnitus, (See Miller TR, Serulle Y, Gandhi D: Arterial abnormalities leading to tinnitus, in this issue.) Even with the narrowed differential diagnosis for tinnitus caused by the venous system, these anomalies are the most commonly encountered cause in the work-up of PST.[2] Hence, it is important that radiologists familiarize themselves with the imaging features of these abnormalities. Potential venous causes of PST include idiopathic intracranial hypertension, sigmoid sinus wall anomalies, transverse and sigmoid sinus stenosis, jugular bulb anomalies, and prominent posterior fossa emissary veins.[2] Idiopathic intracranial hypertension (IIH) is discussed first, and, as noted, there seems to be an overlap of clinical features with patients diagnosed with sigmoid sinus wall anomalies.[3]

IDIOPATHIC INTRACRANIAL HYPERTENSION

IIH, known in the past as benign intracranial hypertension and pseudotumor cerebri, is a disorder primarily affecting obese women in the age range of 20 to 45 years. Its increasing incidence seems to be related to the ever-growing percentage of patients with morbid obesity.[4,5] The most common presenting symptoms are headache, followed by transient visual obscurations, back pain, PST, and visual loss, with approximately 10% of patients developing bilateral blindness.[5]

Disclosures: None.
[a] Neuroradiology Division, Department of Radiology & Medical Imaging, University of Virginia, Charlottesville, VA, USA; [b] Division of Interventional Neuroradiology, Department of Diagnostic Radiology and Nuclear Medicine, University of Maryland School of Medicine, 22 South Greene Street, Baltimore, MD 21201, USA
* Corresponding author. Division of Neuroradiology, Department of Diagnostic Radiology and Nuclear Medicine, University of Maryland School of Medicine, 22 South Greene street, Baltimore, MD 21201.
E-mail address: praghavan@umm.edu

PST is usually bilateral. Papilledema is an important clinical sign on ophthalmoscopic examination, although not necessarily present in all patients. Opening cerebrospinal fluid (CSF) pressure during lumbar puncture is typically greater than 25 cm H_2O. A diagnosis of IIH is made according to the modified Dandy Criteria (Box 1).

Several theories have been proposed to explain the presence of increased CSF pressure in these patients, including increased CSF production, decreased CSF absorption, increased interstitial fluid volume with resultant cerebral edema, and dural sinus stenosis.[4,6] Impairment of CSF absorption and compromise of dural sinus blood flow have been suggested to be interrelated.[7,8] There is still debate as to whether transverse sinus stenosis is the cause or result of IIH. Several reports have shown resolution of stenosis within the transverse dural venous sinus after intracranial pressure normalization via ventriculoperitoneal shunting, lumboperitoneal shunting, or lumbar puncture.[7,9–12] However, there are also reports showing persistent transverse sinus stenosis after normalization of the intracranial pressure.[13] A study using computed tomography (CT) venograms analyzed the morphology of the transverse dural sinus and its adjacent bony grooves in both patients with IIH and control subjects, with results suggesting a varied cause for sinus stenosis, including developmental or fixed narrowing and narrowing caused by compression secondary to increased ICP.[14]

Magnetic resonance (MR) imaging without and with contrast, including MR venogram (MRV), is the study of choice in the work-up for IIH. Orbit-specific sequences can aid in identification of the subtle ocular findings. Imaging findings associated with IIH are outlined in Box 2 and Fig. 1. An interesting association exists between IIH and the presence of spontaneous CSF fistulas. In theory, the persistent increased intracranial pressure leads to the development of prominent arachnoid granulations within the skull base. When these prominent arachnoid granulations develop over pneumatized bone, bony thinning and disruption of the dura can occur.[15] Typical locations for CSF fistulas to develop include the tegmen tympani, floor of the middle cranial fossa, lateral wall of the sphenoid sinus, and cribriform plates.[16] Treatment options for IIH include weight loss/lifestyle modification, medical treatment with carbonic anhydrase inhibitors and inhibitors of growth hormone/insulinlike growth factor 1, CSF diversion, optic nerve sheath fenestration, and endovascular transverse sinus stenting (See: Hui FK, Abruzzo T, Ansari SA. Endovascular Interventions for Idiopathic Intracranial Hypertension and Venous Tinnitus-New Horizons, in this issue) (Fig. 2).[4,17,18]

SIGMOID SINUS WALL ANOMALIES

Sigmoid sinus wall anomalies (SSWAs) are an increasingly recognized diagnosis in the work-up of PST. This spectrum of anomalies includes a thin but intact sigmoid sinus plate, focal dehiscence of the sigmoid sinus plate, diverticulum formation with a focal protrusion of the vascular elements into the mastoid air cells, and ectasia with smooth bulging of the sigmoid sinus into the

---

Box 1
Modified Dandy Criteria for IIH

1. Signs and symptoms of increased intracranial pressure
2. No localizing symptoms on neurologic examination
3. Awake and alert patient
4. Absence of deformity, displacement, or obstruction of the ventricular system
5. No other cause of increased intracranial pressure
6. Normal neuroimaging except for typical findings of increased intracranial pressure

Data from Wall M, Kupersmith MJ, Kieburtz KD, et al. The idiopathic intracranial hypertension treatment trial: clinical profile at baseline. JAMA Neurol 2014;71(6):693–701.

Box2
Imaging features associated with IIH

1. Partially empty sella
2. Distal transverse dural sinus stenosis
3. Small or slitlike lateral and third ventricles
4. Distension and tortuosity of the optic nerve sheath
5. Optic nerve sheath enhancement secondary to venous congestion
6. Posterior globe flattening at the lamina cribrosa
7. Intraocular protrusion of the optic nerve head
8. Dural ectasia
9. Bony thinning and remodeling of the skull base
10. Spontaneous CSF fistulas or meningoencephaloceles

Data from Refs.[6,16,19]

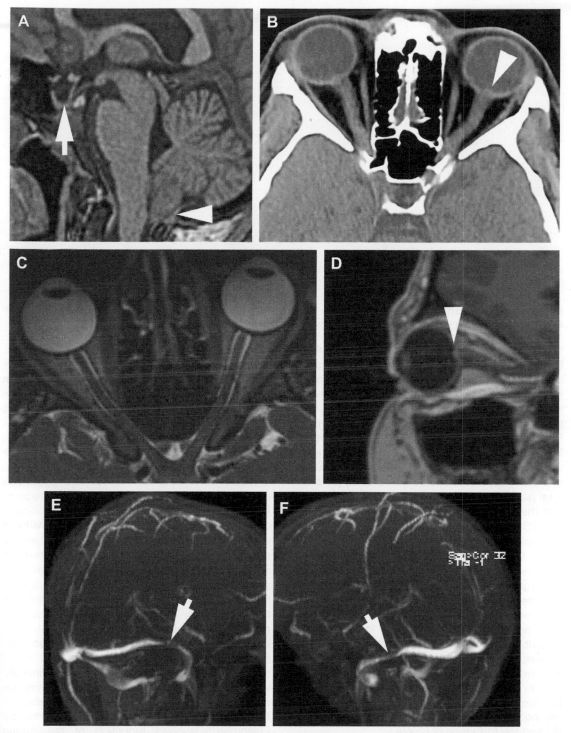

Fig. 1. Findings associated with IIH. (*A*) Sagittal T1 Three Dimensional Magnetization Prepared Rapid Acquisition GRE with a partially empty sella (*arrow*). Note the low-lying cerebellar tonsils with mild crowding at the foramen magnum (*arrowhead*). (*B*) Axial CT with mild tortuosity of the left optic nerve sheath and bilateral protrusion of the optic nerve heads (*arrowhead*). (*C*) Axial high-resolution T2 showing mildly prominent bilateral optic nerve sheaths without significant tortuosity. (*D*) Sagittal T1 postcontrast with intraocular protrusion of the optic nerve head and enhancement at the lamina cribrosa (*arrowhead*). (*E, F*) Maximum intensity projection reformatted images from a time-of-flight MRV showing bilateral stenosis of the distal transverse sinuses (*arrows*).

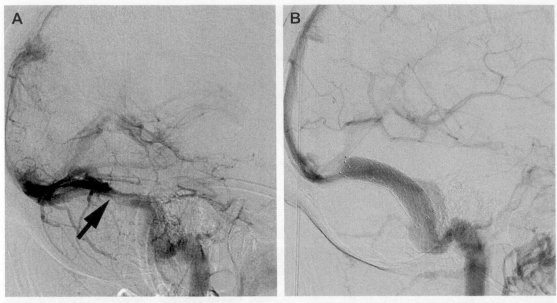

Fig. 2. (A) Venous catheter angiogram showing stenosis in the distal transverse sinus (arrow). (B) Subsequent angiogram following placement of a stent across the stenosis in a patient with IIH.

mastoid air cells without a focal diverticulum. Diverticula can manifest as sessile outpouchings or as narrow-necked, pedunculated structures. It is also possible for more than 1 anomaly to coexist. Several reports have identified SSWA as a common imaging finding in the work-up of PST. The most common abnormality identified by Mattox and Hudgins[2] in the evaluation of patients with constant pulsatile tinnitus was a diverticulum of the lateral surface of the sigmoid sinus (11 of 54 total patients). Schoeff and colleagues[20] reported that the prevalence of SSWA in patients with PST was 23% versus 1.2% in asymptomatic patients. The patients in this study with SSWA were exclusively female, young (mean age of 36.6 years), and presented with objective tinnitus. Harvey and colleagues[3] reported on the demographic features of patients with SSWA showing that most patients were female, between the ages of 25 and 40 years, with an increased body mass index, closely resembling the IIH patient population. These studies suggest a potential association between IIH and SSWA, and a possible explanation for PST in patients with IIH. Further work is needed to elucidate the nature of this association and any potential pathophysiologic mechanism linking IIH and the formation of SSWA.

CT is the study of choice for the evaluation of potential SSWA. CT angiography timed to visualize both arterial and venous structures with temporal bone reconstructions is sensitive in identifying potential abnormalities.[21] CT images should be reconstructed for a high-resolution algorithm with a 0.67-mm section thickness, small field of view, and both axial and coronal reformats provided for analysis. Bone windows must be carefully scrutinized to evaluate the integrity of the sigmoid sinus plate. A typical CT protocol is provided in Table 1. Subtle findings can be difficult to identify, especially in the case of bony dehiscence without diverticulum formation (Figs. 3–5). Eisenman[22] reported several useful signs to use in difficult cases (Box 3).

Treatment options for PST caused by SSWA include surgical and endovascular techniques. A few case reports have described endovascular coil obliteration of a sigmoid diverticulum with or without stenting to avoid coil migration in the successful treatment of PST.[23–25] Transmastoid sigmoid sinus wall reconstruction is an evolving surgical technique gaining increasing popularity for the treatment of SSWA. The reported surgical techniques vary slightly but generally include a postauricular approach, extended mastoidectomy, skeletonization of the sigmoid sinus, and reconstruction of the sigmoid sinus wall to its normal smooth contour with the goal to eliminate vascular turbulence and decrease transmission of vibrations through the mastoid air cells.[22,26] Reconstruction of the sinus wall as reported by Eisenman[22] involves reduction of the ectatic vascular portion with bipolar cautery, extraluminal placement of a soft tissue graft between the dura and posterior fossa bony plate, and bony defect reconstruction with bone cement and/or an outer autologous bone plate (See: Eisenman DJ, Teplitzky TB, Surgical Treatment of Tinnitus, in this issue).[22,27]

Table 1
Protocol for CT of the temporal bone with contrast on a 64 slice CT scanner

	Image Acquisition
Parameter Type	
Thickness/increments (mm)	0.67/0.33
kVp	140
mAs	350
Resolution	High
Collimation	64 × 0.625
Pitch	0.358
Rotation time	0.75
Scan FOV (mm)	200
Reconstruction	0.67-mm slides at 0.33-mm intervals, coronal reformations on 1-mm slides at 1-mm intervals
Scan delay for postcontrast imaging	Automatic image acquisition 20 s after appearance of contrast in common carotid arteries
Contrast	100 mL of Omnipaque iohexol injection GE Healthcare at 1.5 mL/s followed by 50-mL saline flush

Abbreviation: kVp, kilovolt peak.
Courtesy of Tayfor Teplitzky, MD, University of Maryland School of Medicine, Baltimore, MD, USA.

A report by Otto and colleagues[26] described successful resolution of PST in 3 patients with diverticula of the sigmoid sinus after transmastoid reconstruction. Harvey and colleagues[3] reported successful resolution of PST in 30 of 33 patients with either diverticula or dehiscence of the sigmoid sinus following transmastoid reconstruction. A recent article by Raghavan and colleagues[27] reported resolution of PST following transmastoid reconstruction in 11 of 13 patients. The patients in this study all underwent postoperative imaging allowing for analysis of imaging characteristics associated with this innovative surgical technique. Of particular importance is the appearance of the soft tissue graft between the sigmoid sinus and reconstructed bony plate, appearing as low-attenuation material on contrast-enhanced CT with a variable amount of mass effect and narrowing on the adjacent sigmoid sinus, not to be confused with sinus thrombosis (**Fig. 6**). As this procedure grows in popularity radiologists should become familiar with the expected postoperative

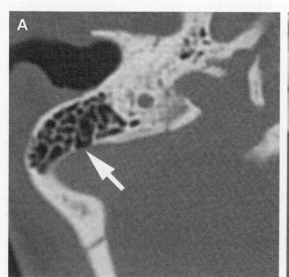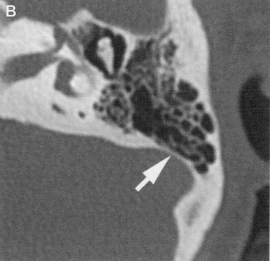

Fig. 3. (*A*) Axial CT showing subtle dehiscence of the sigmoid plate with the air-on-sinus sign (*arrow*). (*B*) CT showing an intact but thin contralateral sigmoid plate (*arrow*).

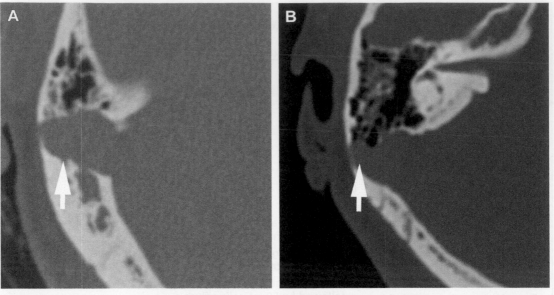

Fig. 4. (A) Axial CT showing a prominent sigmoid sinus diverticulum (arrow) extending though the mastoid air cells to the outer surface of the calvarium. (B) Axial contrast-enhanced CT showing a smaller sigmoid sinus diverticulum (arrow) as a focal outpouching into the mastoid air cells. Note the loss of the normal lateral semicircular contour of the sinus.

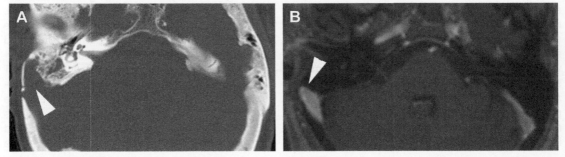

Fig. 5. (A) Axial CT showing a large right sigmoid sinus diverticulum extending anteriorly into opacified mastoid air cells (arrowhead). (B) Axial postcontrast T1 MR imaging showing ectasia of the right sigmoid sinus as a smooth bulging of the sinus into the mastoid air cells without a focal diverticulum (arrowhead).

Box 3
Useful imaging signs in the identification of SSWA

1. Irregularity of the semicircular contour of the bony sigmoid sinus wall

2. Focal thinning of the calvarial cortex adjacent to the sigmoid sinus wall

3. Absence of the thin layer of cortical bone overlying the sinus

4. Air-on-sinus sign: direct contact of the mastoid air cells with the adjacent sinus

Data from Eisenman DJ. Sinus wall reconstruction for sigmoid sinus diverticulum and dehiscence: a standardized surgical procedure for a range of radiographic findings. Otol Neurotol 2011;32(7):1116–9.

---

imaging appearance and any potential complications, including sinus thrombosis.

HIGH-RIDING/DEHISCENT JUGULAR BULB

The jugular bulb is normally separated from the posterior hypotympanum by the bony jugular plate. It receives venous blood from the sigmoid sinus and transmits most of the flow inferiorly to the internal jugular vein.[28,29] The normal superior boundary of the jugular bulb lies below the floor of the hypotympanum, defined as a line connecting the tympanic annulus and base of the cochlear promontory.[30] A high-riding jugular bulb is a normal anatomic variant, more commonly seen on the right, which can be identified on axial CT images when the roof of the bulb is seen at or

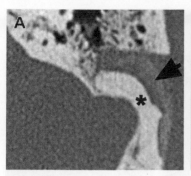
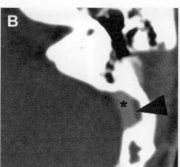
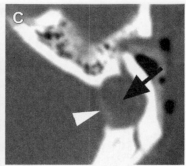

Fig. 6. Postoperative imaging after transmastoid sigmoid sinus wall reconstruction. (*A*) Axial CT in bony algorithm showing the autologous bone pate (*black arrow*) lateral to the well-defined bony cement material (*asterisk*). (*B*) Axial contrast-enhanced CT in soft tissue algorithm showing the normal-appearing soft tissue graft as hypodense material (*black arrowhead*) along the lateral margin of the sigmoid sinus (*asterisk*). (*C*) Axial contrast-enhanced CT showing the edematous soft tissue graft (*black arrow*) causing compression of the sigmoid sinus lumen (*white arrowhead*). (*From* Raghavan P, Serulle Y, Gandhi D, et al. Postoperative imaging findings following sigmoid sinus wall reconstruction for pulse synchronous tinnitus. AJNR Am J Neuroradiol 2016;37(1):136–42; with permission.)

above the same level of the basal turn of the cochlea (**Figs. 7** and **8**).[28] Its recognition is important in the presurgical work-up for lesions in the cerebellopontine angle and internal auditory canal, because inadvertent puncture during translabyrinthine surgery can result in catastrophic hemorrhage.[30] A focal outpouching from the jugular bulb is occasionally identified and is termed a jugular bulb diverticulum. This structure usually protrudes superiorly and medially into the petrous temporal bone and can be associated with sensorineural hearing loss and PST[28,31] The bony jugular plate can be thin or dehiscent **Fig. 8** with or without superior lateral protrusion of the high-riding bulb

into the posterior hypotympanum (see **Fig. 7**). In the case of dehiscent jugular bulb, otoscopy reveals a posterior inferior blue retrotympanic mass. This anomaly is also important to note in order to avoid myringotomy and inadvertent puncture of the vascular structure leading to massive hemorrhage.

POSTERIOR FOSSA EMISSARY VEINS

Emissary veins serve as a communication between the dural venous sinuses and extracranial venous system. Two posterior fossa emissary veins are important to note in the work-up of

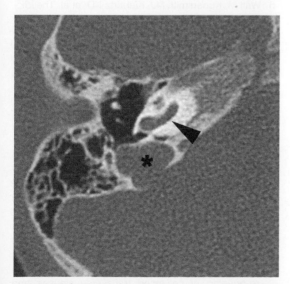

Fig. 7. Axial temporal bone CT showing a high-riding jugular bulb (*asterisk*) extending above the level of the basal turn of the cochlea (*arrowhead*). The thin bony jugular plate is intact between the jugular bulb and middle ear cavity.

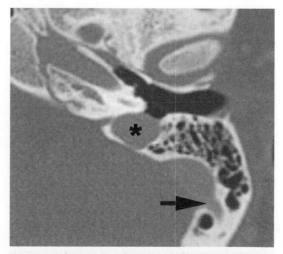

Fig. 8. Axial contrast-enhanced CT showing dehiscence of the jugular plate between the jugular bulb (*asterisk*) and the hypotympanum. Note the origin of a mastoid emissary vein from the sigmoid sinus (*arrow*).

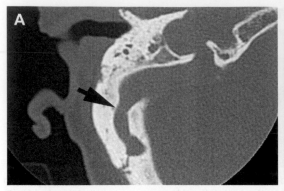
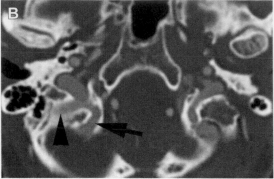

Fig. 9. Posterior fossa emissary veins. (*A*) A mastoid emissary vein extending posteriorly from the posterior portion of the sigmoid sinus (*arrow*). (*B*) A posterior condylar emissary vein (*arrow*) extending posteriorly from the medial distal end of the sigmoid sinus (*arrowhead*).

PST: the posterior condylar emissary vein and the mastoid emissary vein (**Fig. 9**). Mastoid emissary veins course from the midportion of the sigmoid sinus to join extracranial venous structures such as the deep cervical vein or a posterior auricular vein to join the vertebral venous plexus.[32,33] The posterior condylar emissary vein courses from the medial lower end of the sigmoid or marginal sinus to the vertebral venous plexus traveling through the osseous condylar canal in the occipital condyle.[33] Variant venous anatomy, such as a hypoplastic jugular vein, can result in primary dural sinus drainage through an enlarged emissary vein to the vertebral plexus.[34] Emissary veins do not contain valves, which allows bidirectional flow and possible turbulence, a potential cause of tinnitus.[35] Several case reports have shown an association between a dilated posterior fossa emissary vein and PST.[35–38] Treatment options have included endovascular venous embolization, surgical ligation, and observation with lifestyle modification.

SUMMARY

Although there is a limited set of venous abnormalities resulting in PST, they are the most commonly identified diagnosis on imaging. The findings can be subtle and their identification requires meticulous evaluation along with knowledge of the clinical information with regard to laterality and nature of the PST. Knowledge of the clinical profile of each patient also aids in interpretation because there seems to be an association between SSWA and patients with IIH. Many times no distinct abnormality can be identified in the work-up for tinnitus; however, knowledge of potential venous anomalies and reporting them to the referring clinician can greatly aid in the diagnosis and treatment of this often-debilitating disease.

REFERENCES

1. Vattoth S, Shah R, Cure JK. A compartment-based approach for the imaging evaluation of tinnitus. AJNR Am J Neuroradiol 2010;31(2):211–8.
2. Mattox DE, Hudgins P. Algorithm for evaluation of pulsatile tinnitus. Acta Otolaryngol 2008;128(4):427–31.
3. Harvey RS, Hertzano R, Kelman SE, et al. Pulse-synchronous tinnitus and sigmoid sinus wall anomalies: descriptive epidemiology and the idiopathic intracranial hypertension patient population. Otol Neurotol 2014;35(1):7–15.
4. Batra R, Sinclair A. Idiopathic intracranial hypertension; research progress and emerging themes. J Neurol 2014;261(3):451–60.
5. Wall M, Kupersmith MJ, Kieburtz KD, et al. The idiopathic intracranial hypertension treatment trial: clinical profile at baseline. JAMA Neurol 2014;71(6):693–701.
6. Degnan AJ, Levy LM. Pseudotumor cerebri: brief review of clinical syndrome and imaging findings. AJNR Am J Neuroradiol 2011;32:1986–93.
7. Scoffings DJ, Pickard JD, Higgins JN. Resolution of transverse sinus stenoses immediately after CSF withdrawal in idiopathic intracranial hypertension. J Neurol Neurosurg Psychiatry 2007;78(8):911–2.
8. Higgins JN, Cousins C, Owler BK, et al. Idiopathic intracranial hypertension: 12 cases treated by venous sinus stenting. J Neurol Neurosurg Psychiatry 2003;74(12):1662–6.
9. Higgins JN, Pickard JD. Lateral sinus stenoses in idiopathic intracranial hypertension resolving after CSF diversion. Neurology 2004;62(10):1907–8.
10. De Simone R, Marano E, Fiorillo C, et al. Sudden re-opening of collapsed transverse sinuses and longstanding clinical remission after a single lumbar puncture in a case of idiopathic intracranial hypertension. Pathogenetic implications. Neurol Sci 2005;25(6):342–4.

11. Rohr A, Dörner L, Stingele R, et al. Reversibility of venous sinus obstruction in idiopathic intracranial hypertension. AJNR Am J Neuroradiol 2007;28(4): 656–9.

12. McGonigal A, Bone I, Teasdale E. Resolution of transverse sinus stenosis in idiopathic intracranial hypertension after L-P shunt. Neurology 2004; 62(3):514–5.

13. Bono F, Giliberto C, Mastrandrea C, et al. Transverse sinus stenoses persist after normalization of the CSF pressure in IIH. Neurology 2005;65(7):1090–3.

14. Connor SE, Siddiqui MA, Stewart VR, et al. The relationship of transverse sinus stenosis to bony groove dimensions provides an insight into the aetiology of idiopathic intracranial hypertension. Neuroradiology 2008;50(12):999–1004.

15. Schlosser RJ, Woodworth BA, Wilensky EM, et al. Spontaneous cerebrospinal fluid leaks: a variant of benign intracranial hypertension. Ann Otol Rhinol Laryngol 2006;115(7):495–500.

16. Alonso RC, de la Peña MJ, Caicoya AG, et al. Spontaneous skull base meningoencephaloceles and cerebrospinal fluid fistulas. Radiographics 2013; 33(2):553–70.

17. Ahmed RM, Wilkinson M, Parker GD, et al. Transverse sinus stenting for idiopathic intracranial hypertension: a review of 52 patients and of model predictions. AJNR Am J Neuroradiol 2011;32(8): 1408–14.

18. Albuquerque FC, Dashti SR, Hu YC, et al. Intracranial venous sinus stenting for benign intracranial hypertension: clinical indications, technique, and preliminary results. World Neurosurg 2011;75(5–6): 648–52 [discussion: 592–5].

19. Vaghela V, Hingwala DR, Kapilamoorthy TR, et al. Spontaneous intracranial hypo and hypertensions: an imaging review. Neurol India 2011;59(4):506–12.

20. Schoeff S, Nicholas B, Mukherjee S, et al. Imaging prevalence of sigmoid sinus dehiscence among patients with and without pulsatile tinnitus. Otolaryngol Head Neck Surg 2014;150(5):841–6.

21. Krishnan A, Mattox DE, Fountain AJ, et al. CT arteriography and venography in pulsatile tinnitus: preliminary results. AJNR Am J Neuroradiol 2006;27(8): 1635–8.

22. Eisenman DJ. Sinus wall reconstruction for sigmoid sinus diverticulum and dehiscence: a standardized surgical procedure for a range of radiographic findings. Otol Neurotol 2011;32(7):1116–9.

23. Mehanna R, Shaltoni H, Morsi H, et al. Endovascular treatment of sigmoid sinus aneurysm presenting as devastating pulsatile tinnitus. A case report and review of literature. Interv Neuroradiol 2010;16(4): 451–4.

24. Houdart E, Chapot R, Merland JJ. Aneurysm of a dural sigmoid sinus: a novel vascular cause of pulsatile tinnitus. Ann Neurol 2000;48(4):669–71.

25. Sanchez TG, Murao M, de Medeiros IR, et al. A new therapeutic procedure for treatment of objective venous pulsatile tinnitus. Int Tinnitus J 2002;8(1): 54–7.

26. Otto KJ, Hudgins PA, Abdelkafy W, et al. Sigmoid sinus diverticulum: a new surgical approach to the correction of pulsatile tinnitus. Otol Neurotol 2007; 28(1):48–53.

27. Raghavan P, Serulle Y, Gandhi D, et al. Postoperative imaging findings following sigmoid sinus wall reconstruction for pulse synchronous tinnitus. AJNR Am J Neuroradiol 2015. [Epub ahead of print].

28. Ong CK, Fook-Hin Chong V. Imaging of jugular foramen. Neuroimaging Clin North Am 2009;19(3): 469–82.

29. Lo WW, Solti-Bohman LG. High-resolution CT of the jugular foramen: anatomy and vascular variants and anomalies. Radiology 1984;150(3):743–7.

30. Overton SB, Ritter FN. A high placed jugular bulb in the middle ear: a clinical and temporal bone study. Laryngoscope 1973;83(12):1986–91.

31. Presutti L, Laudadio P. Jugular bulb diverticula. ORL J Otorhinolaryngol Relat Spec 1991;53(1):57–60.

32. San Millan Ruiz D, Gailloud P, Rüfenacht DA, et al. The craniocervical venous system in relation to cerebral venous drainage. AJNR Am J Neuroradiol 2002; 23(9):1500–8.

33. Mortazavi MM, Tubbs RS, Riech S, et al. Anatomy and pathology of the cranial emissary veins: a review with surgical implications. Neurosurgery 2012; 70(5):1312–8 [discussion: 1318–9].

34. Hoffmann O, Klingebiel R, Braun JS, et al. Diagnostic pitfall: atypical cerebral venous drainage via the vertebral venous system. AJNR Am J Neuroradiol 2002;23(3):408–11.

35. Lee SH, Kim SS, Sung KY, et al. Pulsatile tinnitus caused by a dilated mastoid emissary vein. J Korean Med Sci 2013;28(4):628–30.

36. Forte V, Turner A, Liu P. Objective tinnitus associated with abnormal mastoid emissary vein. J Otolaryngol 1989;18(5):232–5.

37. Lambert PR, Cantrell RW. Objective tinnitus in association with an abnormal posterior condylar emissary vein. Am J Otol 1986;7(3):204–7.

38. Chauhan NS, Sharma YP, Bhagra T, et al. Persistence of multiple emissary veins of posterior fossa with unusual origin of left petrosquamosal sinus from mastoid emissary. Surg Radiol Anat 2011; 33(9):827–31.

Dural Arteriovenous Fistulae
Imaging and Management

Yafell Serulle, MD, PhD[a], Timothy R. Miller, MD[a],
Dheeraj Gandhi, MBBS, MD[a,b],*

KEYWORDS

• Dural arteriovenous fistula • Tinnitus • Angiography • Endovascular embolization

KEY POINTS

- Intracranial dural arteriovenous fistulae (DAVF) are pathologic shunts between dural arteries to dural veins or a venous sinus and are an important cause of pulsatile tinnitus.
- Digital subtraction angiography allows the accurate characterization and classification of DAVF and remains the gold standard modality for their diagnosis.
- The pattern of venous drainage determines the type and risk of intracranial bleeding of DAVF.
- The goal of treatment is to obliterate the site of the shunt with elimination of retrograde cortical venous drainage.
- Endovascular approach has become a first-line option for treatment of DAVF.

INTRODUCTION

Dural arteriovenous fistulae (DAVF) are abnormal connections between meningeal arteries and dural venous sinuses, meningeal veins, or cortical veins.[1] By definition, DAVF are located within the dura, most frequently on the wall of or immediately around the venous sinuses. They account for approximately 10% to 15% of intracranial arteriovenous shunts and are typically encountered in middle-aged adults with a median age of onset in the sixth decade.[2–4]

Most reported intracranial DAVF involve the transverse and sigmoid sinuses.[5–7] Patients with DAVF involving the transverse and sigmoid sinuses (Fig. 1) often present with ipsilateral retroauricular

pain and pulsatile tinnitus that is usually audible on auscultation of the mastoid area. Pulsatile tinnitus is known to result from nonlaminar blood flow caused by increased blood flow or a reduced vascular cross-sectional area, and is often secondary to an identifiable, vascular anomaly.[8–10] This symptom is associated with approximately 80% of transverse and sigmoid sinus DAVF, which could be explained by direct transmission of the venous bruit to the inner ear through the temporal bone. In addition, intracranial DAVF are the most common cause of objective pulsatile tinnitus in patients with normal otoscopic examination.[2,11,12]

Pulsatile tinnitus is often the only presenting symptom in low-grade DAVF with solely antero-grade venous drainage (Borden type I, discussed

Disclosure: The authors have nothing to disclose.
[a] Division of Interventional Neuroradiology, Department of Diagnostic Radiology, University of Maryland School of Medicine, 22 South Greene Street, Baltimore, MD, USA; [b] Departments of Radiology, Neurology and Neurosurgery, University of Maryland School of Medicine, 22 South Greene Street, Baltimore, MD 21201, USA
* Corresponding author.
E-mail address: dgandhi@umm.edu

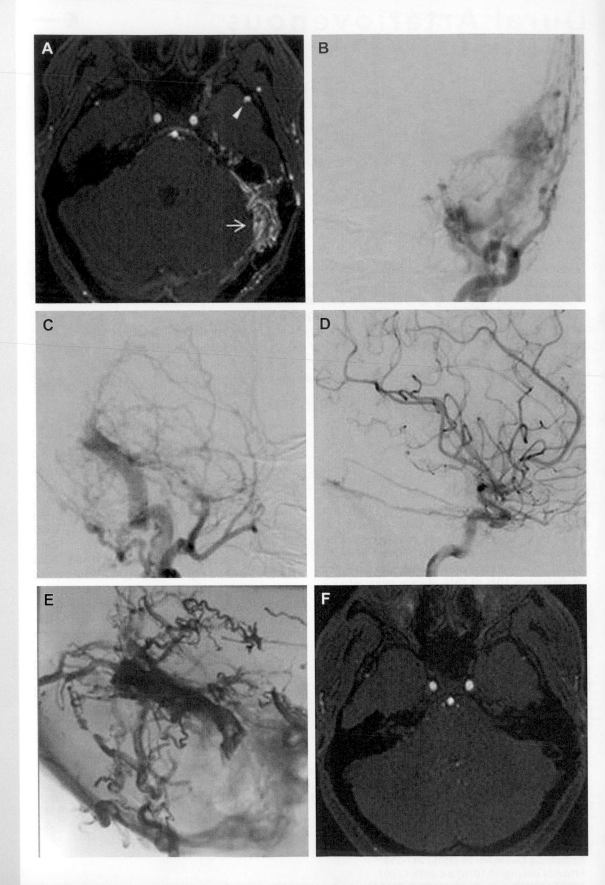

later).[13] The pulsatile tinnitus caused by DAVF can be unbearably loud and can often be heard by the clinician too. The occipital artery often contributes to the blood supply of these lesions and is generally hypertrophied. Compression of the occipital artery against the mastoid process therefore reduces the tinnitus on physical examination.[8]

The causes of DAVF remain incompletely understood. Although in the pediatric population most DAVF are congenital and often associated with structural venous abnormalities, most DAVF are thought to be acquired.[14,15] The development of venous or dural sinus thrombosis and venous hypertension with aberrant angiogenesis has been associated with the pathogenesis of these lesions.[16] The causal role of venous thrombosis is supported by the association of DAVF with hypercoagulable states such as factor V Leiden; hyperhomocysteinemia; and antithrombin, protein C, and protein S deficiencies.[17] The altered angiogenesis leading to DAVF can occur within the dura following an inciting event such as trauma, surgery, chronic Infection, or sinus thrombosis. However, many cases of DAVF are sporadic without any clear inciting event.

The natural history of DAVF varies from spontaneous resolution to fatal hemorrhage, and this do pends to a great extent on their venous drainage patterns.[16,17] Given this large spectrum, it is not the diagnosis but the expected prognosis of the disease that indicates treatment, which makes it mandatory to obtain a proper classification of patients by diagnostic angiography.

CLASSIFICATION

Several classification schemes have been proposed from different aspects of DAVF to grade their risk and natural course. The classifications put forward by Cognard and colleagues[18] and Borden and colleagues[19] are currently the most widely used (Box 1). Both are used in everyday clinical practice and emphasize the

---

Box 1
Classification of intracranial dural arteriovenous fistulae

Borden Classification

I: Venous drainage into dural sinus

II: Venous drainage into dural sinus with cortical venous drainage (CVD)

III: Venous drainage directly into subarachnoid vein (CVD only)

Cognard Classification

I: Venous drainage into dural sinus with normal antegrade flow

IIa: Venous drainage into dural sinus with retrograde flow

IIb: Venous drainage into dural sinus with normal antegrade flow and CVD

IIa + b: Venous drainage into dural sinus with retrograde flow and CVD

III: Venous drainage directly into subarachnoid vein (CVD only)

IV: Venous drainage directly into subarachnoid vein with venous ectasia

V: Venous drainage directly into spinal perimedullary veins

---

venous drainage patterns associated with the fistula.[20] The 3-step Borden classification is simple to apply and categorizes DAVF based on the site of venous drainage (dural sinus vs cortical vein) as well as the absence or presence of cortical venous drainage (CVD).[19] The Cognard classification is more complex and incorporates additional information on the flow direction in the dural sinus (antegrade vs retrograde) as well as the presence or absence of venous ectasia in the involved cortical veins.[18]

Both grading systems highlight the importance of CVD and associated venous drainage pattern to risk

---

Fig. 1. Middle-aged woman with history of left pulsatile tinnitus and intermittent left facial and left neck pain. (*A*) Time-of-flight head magnetic resonance angiography (MRA) shows abnormal vessels centered on the left sigmoid sinus (*arrow*). Note the asymmetrically enlarged dural vessels on the left side as well as an enlarged left middle meningeal artery (*arrowhead*). (*B*) Anteroposterior and (*C*) lateral diagnostic subtraction angiography images following left external carotid artery injections show an extensive dural arteriovenous fistula of the left transverse sigmoid sinus with multiple arterial feeders, including ipsilateral occipital artery, ascending pharyngeal artery, and middle meningeal artery branches. (*D*) Diagnostic subtraction angiography following left internal carotid artery injection, lateral view, shows additional arterial feeders to the fistula arising from the left meningohypophyseal trunk. (*E*) Following a 3-stage treatment, extensive penetration of the DAVF by the Onyx material is noted. There was complete resolution of the symptoms at the time of the angiogram. (*F*) Time-of-flight head MRA performed shortly after the angiogram shown in (*E*) shows interval resolution of previously seen abnormal vessels over the left sigmoid sinus. The patient reported complete resolution of her tinnitus at the time of this MRA.

of hemorrhage and neurologic deficit. The presence of CVD (Borden type II and III, Cognard types IIb–V) is an aggressive feature that places DAVF in a higher risk category. The higher the type in either classification system, the more likely the DAVF is to be symptomatic as a result of venous congestion. In addition, it has been suggested that subdividing lesions with CVD into symptomatic and asymptomatic types may further improve the accuracy of risk stratification, with symptomatic lesions showing significantly higher risk of annual hemorrhage than asymptomatic types.[21]

Although lesions with aggressive features can occur in any intracranial location, the anterior cranial fossa and tentorium seem to have a higher incidence of aggressive lesions, likely because of the higher likelihood of development of CVD caused by the lack of adjacent dural sinuses to provide venous drainage at these sites.[22] Davies and colleagues[23] reported that 69% of hemorrhagic lesions in their series of 102 DAVF occurred either in the anterior cranial fossa or the tentorium, which was a disproportionately high rate given that these two locations accounted for only 18% of the lesions in their study. Other studies have also corroborated these findings.[3,22,24]

IMAGING FINDINGS

Given their wide range of clinical presentations and the lack of specificity of symptoms, the diagnosis of DAVF can be challenging. Nonenhanced computed tomography (CT) and conventional magnetic resonance (MR) imaging can often appear unremarkable with benign DAVF.[25] When symptomatic, the 2 most common presentations of DAVF are intracranial hemorrhage and nonhemorrhagic neurologic manifestations.[11,26] In either case, diagnostic evaluation usually starts with noncontrast head CT and MR imaging.

The patterns of blood distribution detected with noncontrast head CT or MR imaging in patients with intracranial hemorrhage from ruptured DAVF are not specific.[11] The most common pattern of intracranial hemorrhage in ruptured DAVF is intraparenchymal, usually lobar.[27] Subarachnoid hemorrhage (SAH) is less commonly seen, and is most often associated with DAVF with leptomeningeal or pure CVD. Cognard type V has a high propensity for presenting with SAH.[18] Intraventricular hemorrhage may be present as a result of extension of intraparenchymal or subarachnoid hemorrhage. Subdural hematomas are rarely seen, but have been reported in anterior cranial fossa DAVF.[28]

A focused approach in relation to the patient's symptoms and the possible location of the lesion is required when interpreting cross-sectional studies in patients with suspicion of DAVF.[11] With larger fistulae, CT or MR can show prominent vessels or flow voids that may be associated with a dural sinus (Fig. 2). Cross-sectional imaging may also reveal engorged orbital veins and proptosis in cases of cavernous sinus DAVF, and intraosseous serpentine flow voids can be appreciated in anterior condylar DAVF.[29] In addition, MR imaging can provide complementary information that can help evaluate for associated hydrocephalus, other possible causes of pulsatile tinnitus, as well as signal abnormalities secondary to intracranial venous hypertension.[30]

CT angiography (CTA) and MR angiography (MRA) may detect the fistula and can be used to screen patients suspected of harboring DAVF (see Fig. 2). The fistula may appear as prominent vessels associated with the meninges or dural sinus wall. Enlarged feeding arteries, early dural sinus opacification, and prominent draining veins can all be well characterized with CTA and MRA with very good accuracy.[31–33]

Recent advances in imaging technology have allowed the development of time-resolved MRA and CTA, which use the first-pass effect of intravenous contrast to evaluate the dynamics of blood flow in the intracranial circulation. This technique allows the differentiation of arterial and venous phases and permits the better visualization of arteriovenous shunting.[34–36] Time-resolved MRA at 3T has been reported to have a sensitivity and specificity of 100% compared with angiography for the screening, the follow-up, and the posttreatment evaluation of intracranial DAVF.[37] Time-resolved CTA has also been found to be almost equivalent to angiography in diagnosing and classifying intracranial DAVF.[35]

Digital subtraction angiography remains the gold standard to diagnose DAVF. Thanks to its superior spatial and temporal resolution, catheter angiography can clearly characterize both the arterial supply and venous drainage of the fistula, as well as identify important features of the fistula, such as presence of CVD, venous outflow obstruction, and arterial pedicle or venous aneurysms.[17] In addition, catheter angiography is essential for treatment planning, for which a thorough evaluation of all possible arterial feeders and careful depiction of normal and abnormal veins are required.

GENERAL MANAGEMENT

Conservative treatment is often a consideration for patients with low-grade, benign fistulas (Borden I; Cognard I, IIa).[16,17] Spontaneous thrombosis of

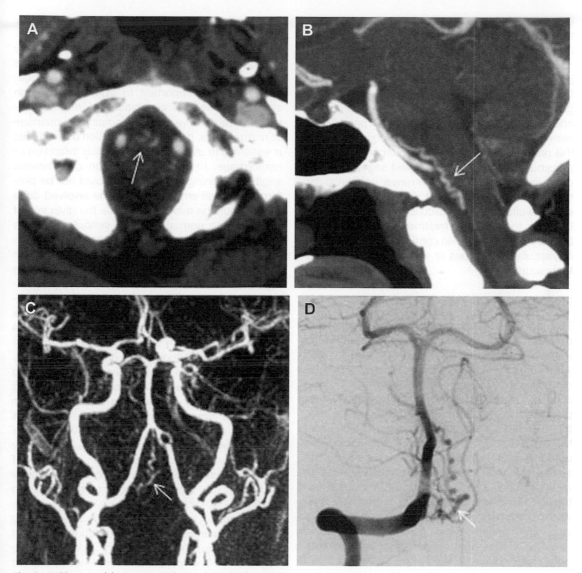

Fig. 2. A 68-year-old woman with incidentally found dural arteriovenous malformation. Axial (*A*) and sagittal (*B*) CT angiogram images show suspicious and prominent vascular structures anterior to the medulla (*arrows*), which raised the suspicion of a vascular malformation. (*C*) Coronal maximal intensity projection of a gadolinium-enhanced MRA shows an abnormal vessel arising from the right vertebral artery, suspicious for a DAVF (*arrow*). (*D*) Digital subtraction angiography shows a DAVF centered on the foramen magnum with arterial supply from small arterial branches arising off the medial aspect of the right vertebral artery and venous drainage via tortuous and dilated perimedullary veins (*arrow*).

DAVF may occasionally occur, more commonly in slow-flow cavernous sinus lesions. Carotid self-compression may help promote resolution of the fistula in a minority of these cases.[38,39] However, patients with benign, low-grade lesions electing conservative management should undergo clinical and imaging follow-up because of the risk of conversion to an aggressive lesion.

In contrast, high-grade, aggressive lesions carry significant mortalities as well as important risk of bleeding and nonhemorrhagic neurologic deficits.[38] Variceal or aneurysmal venous dilatation, leptomeningeal venous drainage, and galenic drainage are significant factors predisposing patients to an aggressive neurologic course.[3,40] The overall rate of hemorrhage from DAVF has been estimated at approximately 1.8%. In patients initially presenting with hemorrhage, the risk of rebleeding within the first 2 weeks following the initial hemorrhage has been estimated at up to 35%.[41,42] Therefore, aggressive DAVF should be treated early to avoid complications. In addition, in low-grade lesions with severe debilitating symptoms, including debilitating pulsatile tinnitus, treatment should be considered to reduce symptoms.

At present available therapeutic options for intracranial DAVF include no treatment, conservative management, endovascular treatment, surgery, a combination of endovascular treatment and surgery, and radiosurgery. In the past, DAVF were treated with surgical disconnection of the pathologic arteriovenous communication and possible resection of the involved segment of the dural sinus.[40] However, with newer endovascular therapies and newer, more navigable microcatheters available, endovascular embolization has become the first-line treatment of DAVF.[16,38,43] Surgery is used either in combination with the endovascular techniques or when the endovascular technique fails.

ENDOVASCULAR TREATMENT

The goal of endovascular therapy is the elimination of the arteriovenous shunt.[16,17,38,44] Note that the pathologic entity of DAVF seems to be located within the wall of dural sinuses, veins, or leptomeningeal veins. The pathophysiologic effect of the shunt is exercised on the venous system. Complete and permanent cure can be achieved only by obliterating all pathologic connections between the arterial and venous side of the lesion. This outcome can be obtained by approaching the site of the shunt through the feeding arteries or by sealing the lumen of the draining venous structures. Partial embolization may temporarily alleviate symptoms, but is unlikely to result in a long-term cure. In addition, partial occlusion could negatively alter the venous drainage pattern, potentially inducing CVD.[45]

EMBOLIZATION ACCESS ROUTES

The optimal endovascular approach for treatment of DAVF remains a highly debated and controversial topic. Transarterial, transvenous, and sometimes combined approaches have been used to successfully treat DAVF. A consideration of the advantages and disadvantages of each approach should be given in each case before proceeding with embolization.

Transvenous Embolization

In contrast with brain arteriovenous malformations, venous occlusion is feasible and in many cases highly effective for DAVF (Fig. 3). Transvenous embolization is performed by retrograde catheterization of the involved cortical vein or dural sinus with a microcatheter, which is then subsequently closed by placement of detachable microcoils or liquid embolic agents.[16,46] Permanent and complete sacrifice of a dural sinus may be done while avoiding venous infarction only if the involved sinus does not drain the brain tissue. Therefore, it is important to obtain a thorough study of the venous circulation before embolization.[16] If the dural venous sinus maintains drainage of normal veins, precise identification of the fistula is essential to avoid potential venous infarction or hemorrhage. In general, occlusion of a venous segment draining brain tissue should not be performed. Partial embolization of the involved dural sinus should be avoided because the diversion of flow into the normal cerebral venous pathways can ultimately worsen CVD and convert an originally benign venous pattern to a more aggressive one by blocking its antegrade outlet and forcing high-pressure arterial blood into the retrograde direction or, even worse, into cortical veins.[47]

Benefits of the transvenous approach include the simplicity of retrograde venous access to the fistulous site and the ability to close the shunt in a single session. Although it is difficult to obliterate multiple arteriovenous connections via the feeding arteries, this can easily be achieved by packing the lumen of the single venous channel of the lesion. Therefore, transvenous embolization is the preferred approach when treating DAVF that are supplied by multiple arterial pedicles, which may make a transarterial approach difficult. Rates of complete fistula obliteration using a transvenous technique are high, with reports ranging from 71% to 87%.[48–51]

Cavernous sinus DAVF are particularly amenable to transvenous embolization, with high rates of successful lesion closure (see Fig. 3).[52–54] The ipsilateral inferior petrosal sinus provides the most convenient access to the cavernous sinus. When the ipsilateral inferior petrosal sinus is not found or not accessible, the cavernous sinus might be catheterized via the contralateral inferior petrosal sinus into the contralateral cavernous sinus and then crossing the midline via the intercavernous veins.[55] Other approaches to the cavernous sinus include the facial and superior ophthalmic veins.[52,53,56,57] Direct percutaneous puncture of the cavernous sinus or an orbital vein has also been reported when other venous access routes are unavailable.[52,53,56,57] Overall, the technique is well tolerated, although cavernous sinus embolization may result in cranial neuropathies or worsening of the venous drainage pattern when fistula closure is incomplete.[46]

Risks associated with transvenous embolization of DAVF include vessel perforation, infarction, intracranial hemorrhage, and transient or permanent neurologic deficits related to changes in venous drainage.[16] Other complications include cranial nerve palsies and hearing loss.[48] Recurrence of DAVF in a different location following transvenous embolization of cavernous sinus has been reported.[58–60] Some DAVF cannot be assessed through the venous system, have isolated sinus involvement, or have no sinus involvement. In these cases, a transvenous treatment is not possible.

Transarterial Embolization

The transarterial approach has become a widely used technique to obliterate DAVF. In this technique, the arterial microcatheter must be wedged close to the fistula site to allow the slow push of the liquid embolic agent through the fistula into the proximal venous outlet (Fig. 4).[16,61] If the embolization is too proximal, it can result in persistent arterial shunting and recruitment of collateral flow, whereas if the embolization is too distal it may result in venous occlusion and infarction.

Transarterial embolization of DAVF is typically performed with liquid embolic agents, such as N-butyl-cyanoacrylate (nBCA) or Onyx. Outcomes with this approach have been very favorable. Nelson and colleagues[62] first reported an excellent occlusion rate using arterial embolization with nBCA, with 23 of 23 lesions completely occluded using their proposed wedged microcatheter technique. Their treatment consisted of closing segments of a lesion with nBCA or polyvinyl acetate (PVA) particles to decrease competing inflow followed by a wedged microcatheter injection of nBCA to seal the dural vascular connections.

The transarterial route may not always be feasible because of multiple, small, and tortuous feeders. High-flow fistulas present a particular challenge to transarterial embolization because of the rapid transition from arterial to venous flow across the fistulous point. This rapid transition can result in the passage of even concentrated or high-density liquid embolic material into the venous circulation without occlusion of the connection.[63] To circumvent this problem, balloon occlusion or coil embolization of the feeding artery may be attempted, or, alternatively, balloon and coil embolization of the venous outflow can be performed before injection of the liquid embolic agents.[64]

EMBOLIC AGENTS

Endovascular obliteration of DAVF can be accomplished using a variety of embolic agents, including particles, coils, ethanol, nBCA, and Onyx.[41,54,65,66] Coils have been used successfully in transvenous embolization.[62] When used in a transarterial approach, they are for the most part used as an adjunct to liquid embolic agents to reduce the rate of shunt in high-flow lesions but are rarely curative when used alone.[16] For example, coils can be placed in the venous pouch located close to the fistula and draining only the fistula to attain flow control, along with systemic hypotension during nBCA injection. Coils can also be placed in the feeding artery to reduce flow.[67] Embolization of external carotid artery branches with particles can be easily performed and has been used to reduce shunt flow. However, particulate embolization typically is not curative.[68] Complete obliteration is not likely achieved with this method because some feeding arteries cannot be catheterized and because of the recruitment of blood supply from collateral arteries.[69]

nBCA is a liquid embolic agent that has been extensively used in the treatment of DAVF, mostly using a transarterial approach, with fairly good results.[66] It is injected in liquid form and polymerizes quickly in an ionic environment such as blood. Lipiodol, a radiopaque oil, is added to provide radiopacity and to regulate solidification time.[70,71] One major disadvantage of nBCA is the requirement of a short injection time, usually within minutes. In addition, the appropriate concentration of nBCA needs to be determined, which requires a highly experienced operator.[72] Limited amount of nBCA mixture injection can lead to insufficient embolization and lower cure rate.[62,66,73]

Another concern is the difficulty of controlling nBCA flow after injection, which can result in proximal arterial occlusion in cases of a highly concentrated nBCA or migration to a draining vein in low-concentrated nBCA, which can result in venous infarction or hemorrhage.[72] Although several studies have shown excellent cure rates with the use of nBCA, multiple procedures are often necessary and more than 1 treatment modality may be required for complex lesions.[16,54,74]

Onyx is a more recently developed nonadhesive liquid embolic agent. It is supplied in ready-to-use vials and consists of ethylene-vinyl alcohol copolymer dissolved in various concentrations of dimethylsulfoxide with micronized tantalum powder for radiopacity. Following contact with blood, Onyx gets precipitated and occludes the vessels but is nonadherent to the vessel wall. It allows a slow injection, which allows the operator to control and optimize the amount of artery-to-artery embolization with better penetration of the vascular bed compared with nBCA.[75] Another technical advantage of Onyx is the possibility of performing arteriography in the pauses of 30 to 120 seconds to evaluate residual shunts in dural leaflets and the normal vessels as the lesion is occluded.[76]

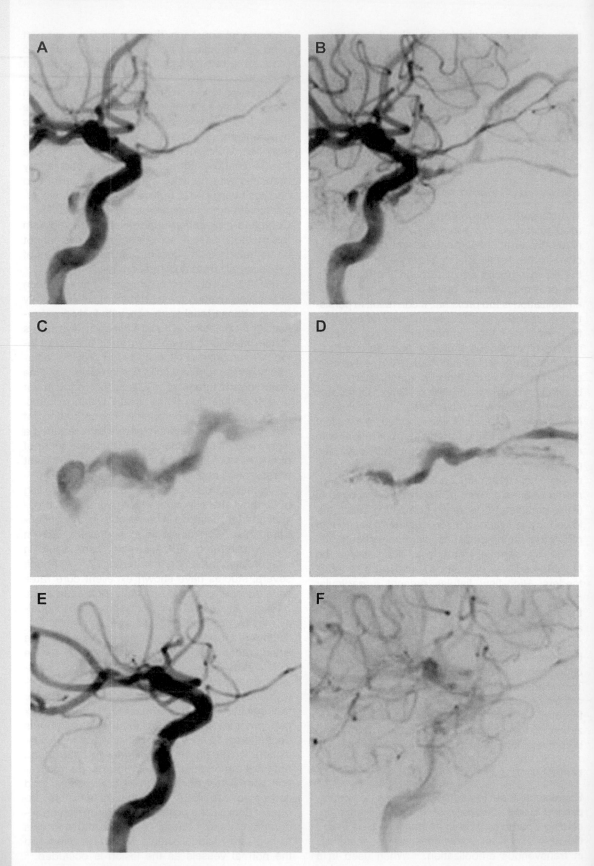

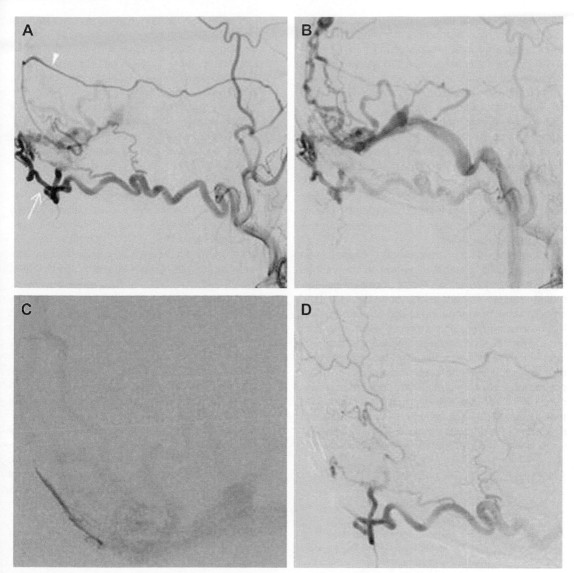

Fig. 4. A 66-year-old man with a history of sudden onset of decreased left lower quadrant vision. Head CT showed a right occipital hemorrhage. (*A*) Early and (*B*) late arterial phases of a right external carotid artery digital subtraction angiogram show a complex paratorcular occipital dural arteriovenous fistula supplied by multiple branches of the right occipital artery (*arrow*) and right middle meningeal artery (*arrowhead*). There is a venous pouch and retrograde cortical reflux as well as venous drainage into the right transverse sinus. (*C*) Selective catheterization of the right middle meningeal artery confirmed arterial supply to the pouch of the dural arteriovenous fistula. Onyx was then injected through the microcatheter and into the fistula. (*D*) Post-Onyx embolization right external carotid artery angiography shows complete occlusion of the fistula with no residual arteriovenous shunting.

Fig. 3. A 70-year-old man with a history of diplopia, right proptosis, conjunctival erythema, and ecchymosis. Early (*A*) and late (*B*) arterial phases of a right internal carotid artery angiogram show a right carotid cavernous fistula supplied predominantly by the inferolateral trunk and meningohypophyseal trunk branches of the right internal carotid artery. The arteriovenous shunting is to the right cavernous sinus, with venous drainage into the superior ophthalmic vein. (*C*) Selective catheterization and injection of the right superior ophthalmic vein shows the microcatheter tip located within the cavernous sinus. (*D*) Multiple platinum microcoils were deployed through the microcatheter and into the cavernous sinus. Postembolization angiography (*E* and *F*) shows complete occlusion of the cavernous-carotid fistula with no significant residual filling.

Excellent cure rates have been reported with this agent, and a high proportion of treatments have been completed in a single session.[65,77] Relative to nBCA, Onyx has been shown to have higher efficacy in initial and durable occlusion rates for embolization of cranial DAVF, while keeping a similar low risk of complications.[76]

Onyx is commercially available in the United States in 2 concentrations of increasing viscosity: 18 or 34 cP. The lower viscosity Onyx 18 may be the preferred agent for plexiform shunt configurations, whereas the Onyx 34 is more suited for large, higher flow fistulas.[11] The Onyx preparation must be shaken for at least 20 minutes before injection in order to obtain homogeneous consistency and opacity.[78]

Complications in transarterial embolization include embolic material migration to the venous site, which may result in venous occlusion exacerbating venous hypertension, catheter retention, embolization of normal vascular structures, and failed or incomplete embolization, which may limit access for future procedures. However, with careful attention to technique and continued improvement of endovascular techniques and materials, major complications of treatment are uncommon and cure rates are excellent. It must be emphasized that these lesions are complex and the treatment modality for a particular patient should always be chosen with multidisciplinary involvement.

REFERENCES

1. Aminoff MJ. Vascular anomalies in the intracranial dura mater. Brain 1973;96:601–12.
2. Lasjaunias P, Chiu M, ter Brugge K, et al. Neurological manifestations of intracranial dural arteriovenous malformations. J Neurosurg 1986;64:724–30.
3. Awad IA, Little JR, Akarawi WP, et al. Intracranial dural arteriovenous malformations: factors predisposing to an aggressive neurological course. J Neurosurg 1990;72:839–50.
4. Houser OW, Campbell JK, Campbell RJ, et al. Arteriovenous malformation affecting the transverse dural venous sinus–an acquired lesion. Mayo Clin Proc 1979;54:651–61.
5. Fermand M, Reizine D, Melki JP, et al. Long term follow-up of 43 pure dural arteriovenous fistulae (AVF) of the lateral sinus. Neuroradiology 1987;29:348–53.
6. Houdart E, Gobin YP, Casasco A, et al. A proposed angiographic classification of intracranial arteriovenous fistulae and malformations. Neuroradiology 1993;35:381–5.
7. Levrier O, Metellus P, Fuentes S, et al. Use of a self-expanding stent with balloon angioplasty in the treatment of dural arteriovenous fistulas involving the transverse and/or sigmoid sinus: functional and neuroimaging-based outcome in 10 patients. J Neurosurg 2006;104:254–63.
8. Hofmann E, Behr R, Neumann-Haefelin T, et al. Pulsatile tinnitus: Imaging and differential diagnosis. Dtsch Arztebl Int 2013;110:451–8.
9. Liyanage SH, Singh A, Savundra P, et al. Pulsatile tinnitus. J Laryngol Otol 2006;120:93–7.
10. Sonmez G, Basekim CC, Ozturk E, et al. Imaging of pulsatile tinnitus: a review of 74 patients. Clin Imaging 2007;31:102–8.
11. Hacein-Bey L, Konstas AA, Pile-Spellman J. Natural history, current concepts, classification, factors impacting endovascular therapy, and pathophysiology of cerebral and spinal dural arteriovenous fistulas. Clin Neurol Neurosurg 2014;121:64–75.
12. Waldvogel D, Mattle HP, Sturzenegger M, et al. Pulsatile tinnitus–a review of 84 patients. J Neurol 1998;245:137–42.
13. Spittau B, Millan DS, El-Sherifi S, et al. Dural arteriovenous fistulas of the hypoglossal canal: systematic review on imaging anatomy, clinical findings, and endovascular management. J Neurosurg 2015;122:883–903.
14. Chaudhary MY, Sachdev VP, Cho SH, et al. Dural arteriovenous malformation of the major venous sinuses: an acquired lesion. AJNR Am J Neuroradiol 1982;3:13–9.
15. Lawton MT, Jacobowitz R, Spetzler RF. Redefined role of angiogenesis in the pathogenesis of dural arteriovenous malformations. J Neurosurg 1997;87:267–74.
16. Gandhi D, Chen J, Pearl M, et al. Intracranial dural arteriovenous fistulas: classification, imaging findings, and treatment. AJNR Am J Neuroradiol 2012;33:1007–13.
17. Miller TR, Gandhi D. Intracranial dural arteriovenous fistulae: clinical presentation and management strategies. Stroke 2015;46:2017–25.
18. Cognard C, Gobin YP, Pierot L, et al. Cerebral dural arteriovenous fistulas: clinical and angiographic correlation with a revised classification of venous drainage. Radiology 1995;194:671–80.
19. Borden JA, Wu JK, Shucart WA. A proposed classification for spinal and cranial dural arteriovenous fistulous malformations and implications for treatment. J Neurosurg 1995;82:166–79.
20. Davies MA, Saleh J, Ter Brugge K, et al. The natural history and management of intracranial dural arteriovenous fistulae. Part 1: benign lesions. Interv Neuroradiol 1997;3:295–302.
21. Zipfel GJ, Shah MN, Refai D, et al. Cranial dural arteriovenous fistulas: modification of angiographic classification scales based on new natural history data. Neurosurg Focus 2009;26:E14.
22. Malik GM, Pearce JE, Ausman JI, et al. Dural arteriovenous malformations and intracranial hemorrhage. Neurosurgery 1984;15:332–9.

23. Davies MA, TerBrugge K, Willinsky R, et al. The validity of classification for the clinical presentation of intracranial dural arteriovenous fistulas. J Neurosurg 1996;85:830–7.

24. Lawton MT, Sanchez-Mejia RO, Pham D, et al. Tentorial dural arteriovenous fistulae: operative strategies and microsurgical results for six types. Neurosurgery 2008;62:110–24 [discussion: 124–5].

25. Noguchi K, Kuwayama N, Kubo M, et al. Intracranial dural arteriovenous fistula with retrograde cortical venous drainage: use of susceptibility-weighted imaging in combination with dynamic susceptibility contrast imaging. AJNR Am J Neuroradiol 2010;31:1903–10.

26. Signorelli F, Della Pepa GM, Sabatino G, et al. Diagnosis and management of dural arteriovenous fistulas: a 10 years single-center experience. Clin Neurol Neurosurg 2015;128:123–9.

27. Cordonnier C, Al-Shahi Salman R, Bhattacharya JJ, et al. Differences between intracranial vascular malformation types in the characteristics of their presenting haemorrhages: prospective, population-based study. J Neurol Neurosurg Psychiatry 2008; 79:47–51.

28. Agid R, Terbrugge K, Rodesch G, et al. Management strategies for anterior cranial fossa (ethmoidal) dural arteriovenous fistulas with an emphasis on endovascular treatment. J Neurosurg 2009;110:79–84.

29. Tanoue S, Kiyosue H, Okahara M, et al. Para-cavernous sinus venous structures: anatomic variations and pathologic conditions evaluated on fat-suppressed 3D fast gradient-echo MR images. AJNR Am J Neuroradiol 2006;27:1083–9.

30. McDougall CG, Halbach VV, Dowd CF, et al. Dural arteriovenous fistulas of the marginal sinus. AJNR Am J Neuroradiol 1997;18:1565–72.

31. Chen JC, Tsuruda JS, Halbach VV. Suspected dural arteriovenous fistula: results with screening MR angiography in seven patients. Radiology 1992; 183:265–71.

32. Noguchi K, Melhem ER, Kanazawa T, et al. Intracranial dural arteriovenous fistulas: evaluation with combined 3D time-of-flight MR angiography and MR digital subtraction angiography. AJR Am J Roentgenol 2004;182:183–90.

33. Narvid J, Do HM, Blevins NH, et al. CT angiography as a screening tool for dural arteriovenous fistula in patients with pulsatile tinnitus: feasibility and test characteristics. AJNR Am J Neuroradiol 2011;32:446–53.

34. Pekkola J, Kangasniemi M. Posterior fossa dural arteriovenous fistulas: diagnosis and follow-up with time-resolved imaging of contrast kinetics (tricks) at 1.5T. Acta Radiol 2011;52:442–7.

35. Willems PW, Brouwer PA, Barfett JJ, et al. Detection and classification of cranial dural arteriovenous fistulas using 4D-CT angiography: initial experience. AJNR Am J Neuroradiol 2011;32:49–53.

36. Meckel S, Maier M, Ruiz DS, et al. MR angiography of dural arteriovenous fistulas: diagnosis and follow-up after treatment using a time-resolved 3D contrast-enhanced technique. AJNR Am J Neuroradiol 2007;28:877–84.

37. Farb RI, Agid R, Willinsky RA, et al. Cranial dural arteriovenous fistula: diagnosis and classification with time-resolved MR angiography at 3T. AJNR Am J Neuroradiol 2009;30:1546–51.

38. Rammos S, Bortolotti C, Lanzino G. Endovascular management of intracranial dural arteriovenous fistulae. Neurosurg Clin North Am 2014;25:539–49.

39. Sarma D, ter Brugge K. Management of intracranial dural arteriovenous shunts in adults. Eur J Radiol 2003;46:206–20.

40. Webb S, Hopkins LN. Intracranial dural arteriovenous fistulas: a treatment paradigm in flux. World Neurosurg 2013;80:47–9.

41. Cognard C, Januel AC, Silva NA Jr, et al. Endovascular treatment of intracranial dural arteriovenous fistulas with cortical venous drainage: new management using Onyx. AJNR Am J Neuroradiol 2008;29:235–41.

42. Duffau H, Lopes M, Janosevic V, et al. Early rebleeding from intracranial dural arteriovenous fistulas: report of 20 cases and review of the literature. J Neurosurg 1999;90:78–84.

43. Chung SJ, Kim JS, Kim JC, et al. Intracranial dural arteriovenous fistulas: analysis of 60 patients. Cerebrovasc Dis 2002;13:79–88.

44. Kobayashi A, Al-Shahi Salman R. Prognosis and treatment of intracranial dural arteriovenous fistulae: a systematic review and meta-analysis. Int J Stroke 2014;9:670–7.

45. De Keukeleire K, Vanlangenhove P, Kalala Okito JP, et al. Transarterial embolization with Onyx for treatment of intracranial non-cavernous dural arteriovenous fistula with or without cortical venous reflux. J Neurointerv Surg 2011;3:224–8.

46. Elhammady MS, Wolfe SQ, Farhat H, et al. Onyx embolization of carotid-cavernous fistulas. J Neurosurg 2010;112:589–94.

47. Davies MA, Ter Brugge K, Willinsky R, et al. The natural history and management of intracranial dural arteriovenous fistulae. Part 2: aggressive lesions. Interv Neuroradiol 1997;3:303–11.

48. Roy D, Raymond J. The role of transvenous embolization in the treatment of intracranial dural arteriovenous fistulas. Neurosurgery 1997;40:1133–41 [discussion: 1141–4].

49. Urtasun F, Biondi A, Casaco A, et al. Cerebral dural arteriovenous fistulas: percutaneous transvenous embolization. Radiology 1996;199:209–17.

50. Yoshida K, Melake M, Oishi H, et al. Transvenous embolization of dural carotid cavernous fistulas: a series of 44 consecutive patients. AJNR Am J Neuroradiol 2010;31:651–5.

51. Jung C, Kwon BJ, Kwon OK, et al. Intraosseous cranial dural arteriovenous fistula treated with transvenous embolization. AJNR Am J Neuroradiol 2009; 30:1173–7.

52. Cheng KM, Chan CM, Cheung YL. Transvenous embolisation of dural carotid-cavernous fistulas by multiple venous routes: a series of 27 cases. Acta Neurochir 2003;145:17–29.

53. Klisch J, Huppertz HJ, Spetzger U, et al. Transvenous treatment of carotid cavernous and dural arteriovenous fistulae: results for 31 patients and review of the literature. Neurosurgery 2003;53:836–56 [discussion: 856–7].

54. Kiyosue H, Hori Y, Okahara M, et al. Treatment of intracranial dural arteriovenous fistulas: current strategies based on location and hemodynamics, and alternative techniques of transcatheter embolization. Radiographics 2004;24:1637–53.

55. Halbach VV, Higashida RT, Hieshima GB, et al. Transvenous embolization of dural fistulas involving the cavernous sinus. AJNR Am J Neuroradiol 1989;10:377–83.

56. Biondi A, Milea D, Cognard C, et al. Cavernous sinus dural fistulae treated by transvenous approach through the facial vein: report of seven cases and review of the literature. AJNR Am J Neuroradiol 2003; 24:1240–6.

57. White JB, Layton KF, Evans AJ, et al. Transorbital puncture for the treatment of cavernous sinus dural arteriovenous fistulas. AJNR Am J Neuroradiol 2007;28:1415–7.

58. Kawaguchi T, Kawano T, Kaneko Y, et al. Dural arteriovenous fistula of the transverse sigmoid sinus after transvenous embolization of the carotid cavernous fistula. No To Shinkei 1999;51:1065–9 [in Japanese].

59. Kubota Y, Ueda T, Kaku Y, et al. Development of a dural arteriovenous fistula around the jugular valve after transvenous embolization of cavernous dural arteriovenous fistula. Surg Neurol 1999;51:174–6.

60. Nakagawa H, Kubo S, Nakajima Y, et al. Shifting of dural arteriovenous malformation from the cavernous sinus to the sigmoid sinus to the transverse sinus after transvenous embolization. A case of left spontaneous carotid-cavernous sinus fistula. Surg Neurol 1992;37:30–8.

61. McConnell KA, Tjoumakaris SI, Allen J, et al. Neuroendovascular management of dural arteriovenous malformations. Neurosurg Clin North Am 2009;20:431–9.

62. Nelson PK, Russell SM, Woo HH, et al. Use of a wedged microcatheter for curative transarterial embolization of complex intracranial dural arteriovenous fistulas: indications, endovascular technique, and outcome in 21 patients. J Neurosurg 2003;98: 498–506.

63. Vanlandingham M, Fox B, Hoit D, et al. Endovascular treatment of intracranial dural arteriovenous fistulas. Neurosurgery 2014;74(Suppl 1):S42–9.

64. Andreou A, Ioannidis I, Nasis N. Transarterial balloon-assisted glue embolization of high-flow arteriovenous fistulas. Neuroradiology 2008;50:267–72.

65. Nogueira RG, Dabus G, Rabinov JD, et al. Preliminary experience with Onyx embolization for the treatment of intracranial dural arteriovenous fistulas. AJNR Am J Neuroradiol 2008;29:91–7.

66. Guedin P, Gaillard S, Boulin A, et al. Therapeutic management of intracranial dural arteriovenous shunts with leptomeningeal venous drainage: report of 53 consecutive patients with emphasis on transarterial embolization with acrylic glue. J Neurosurg 2010;112:603–10.

67. Paramasivam S, Toma N, Niimi Y, et al. Development, clinical presentation and endovascular management of congenital intracranial pial arteriovenous fistulas. J Neurointerv Surg 2013;5:184–90.

68. Gupta A, Periakaruppan A. Intracranial dural arteriovenous fistulas: a review. Indian J Radiol Imaging 2009;19:43–8.

69. Kawaguchi S, Sakaki T, Morimoto T, et al. Surgery for dural arteriovenous fistula in superior sagittal sinus and transverse sigmoid sinus. J Clin Neurosci 2000;7(Suppl 1):47–9.

70. Cromwell LD, Kerber CW. Modification of cyanoacrylate for therapeutic embolization: preliminary experience. AJR Am J Roentgenol 1979;132:799–801.

71. Bank WO, Kerber CW, Cromwell LD. Treatment of intracerebral arteriovenous malformations with isobutyl 2-cyanoacrylate: initial clinical experience. Radiology 1981;139:609–16.

72. Luo CB, Chang FC, Teng MM. Update of embolization of intracranial dural arteriovenous fistula. J Chin Med Assoc 2014;77:610–7.

73. Kim DJ, Willinsky RA, Krings T, et al. Intracranial dural arteriovenous shunts: transarterial glue embolization–experience in 115 consecutive patients. Radiology 2011;258:554–61.

74. Halbach VV, Higashida RT, Hieshima GB, et al. Treatment of dural fistulas involving the deep cerebral venous system. AJNR Am J Neuroradiol 1989; 10:393–9.

75. Gemmete JJ, Ansari SA, McHugh J, et al. Embolization of vascular tumors of the head and neck. Neuroimaging Clin North Am 2009;19:181–98.

76. Rabinov JD, Yoo AJ, Ogilvy CS, et al. Onyx versus n-BCA for embolization of cranial dural arteriovenous fistulas. J Neurointerv Surg 2013;5:306–10.

77. Stiefel MF, Albuquerque FC, Park MS, et al. Endovascular treatment of intracranial dural arteriovenous fistulae using Onyx: a case series. Neurosurgery 2009;65:132–9 [discussion: 139–40].

78. Pierot L, Januel AC, Herbreteau D, et al. Endovascular treatment of brain arteriovenous malformations using Onyx: preliminary results of a prospective multicenter study. Interv Neuroradiol 2005;11:159–64.

Paragangliomas of the Head and Neck

Sean Woolen, MD[a], Joseph J. Gemmete, MD, FACR, FSIR[a,b,c],*

KEYWORDS

- Computed tomography • DOPA-PET • FDG-PET • MR imaging • In 111-DTPA-D-Phe1-octreotide
- I-123 Metaiodobenzylguanidine (MIBG) • Paraganglioma • Pheochromocytoma

KEY POINTS

- The most common paraganglioma locations of the head and neck are the carotid body, jugular, tympanic, and vagal paragangliomas.
- Syndromes associated with a high incidence of paragangliomas include multiple endocrine neoplasia type II, von Hippel-Lindau disease, and neurofibromatosis type I.
- All patients, including those with a sporadic tumor, should be referred for a genetic consultation.
- Jugular and tympanic paragangliomas commonly present with tinnitus and hearing loss, whereas carotid body and vagal paragangliomas usually present with nonpainful palpable neck mass.

INTRODUCTION

Paragangliomas make up a family of neoplasms that develop from the paraganglia tissues, which are themselves of neural crest origin and have similar functions and histologic appearances.[1] They may occur along the ganglia's pathway of embryologic migration extending from the skull base to the pelvic floor.[2] Paraganglia play an important role in organismic hemostasis by acting directly as chemoreceptors or by the secretion of catecholamines in response to stess.[1] Paragangliomas of the head and neck are rare vascular skull-base tumors derived from the paraganglionic system with an estimated incidence of 1:30,000, accounting for 3% of all paragangliomas.[2–4]

The most common paraganglioma locations of the head and neck in descending order are the carotid body, jugular, tympanic, and vagal paragangliomas.[5] Tympanic paragangliomas are the most common primary neoplasms of the middle ear.[6] Jugular paragangliomas are the most common tumor of the jugular foramen.[7] Of the different paraganglioma locations, jugulartympanic are the most common paraganglioma causing tinnitus with incidence of 1 per 1.3 million people per year.[4]

Paragangliomas can be sporadic or familial, with genetic mutations occurring in the SDHB, SDHC, or SDHD genes.[8–10] It is now known that at least 30% of patients with a paraganglioma and no other know risk factors harbor a genetic mutation that increases their risk for these tumors and for other neoplasia.[11] Moreover, other genes discovered within the past 5 years: SDHAF2, TMEM127, MAX, EGLN1, HIF2A, KIF1B, and SDHA, add to the genetic complexity of hereditary paraganglioma-pheochromocytoma syndrome.[11] Sporadic paragangliomas are more common in women, with the average age at presentation of 40 to 50 years, as familial present earlier and more commonly in men.[12] Classic tumor syndromes associated with a high incidence of

Disclosures: None.
[a] Department of Radiology, University of Michigan Health System, Ann Arbor, MI, USA; [b] Department of Neurosurgery, University of Michigan Health System, Ann Arbor, MI, USA; [c] Department of Otolaryngology, University of Michigan Health System, Ann Arbor, MI, USA
* Corresponding author. Department of Radiology, University of Michigan Health System, UH B1D 328, 1500 East Medical Center Drive, Ann Arbor, MI 48109-5030.
E-mail address: gemmete@med.umich.edu

Neuroimag Clin N Am 26 (2016) 259–278
http://dx.doi.org/10.1016/j.nic.2015.12.005
1052-5149/16/$ – see front matter © 2016 Elsevier Inc. All rights reserved.

paragangliomas included multiple endocrine neoplasia type II (MEN II), von Hippel-Lindau (VHL) disease, and neurofibromatosis type I (NF I).[13] Multicentric paragangliomas occur in 10% to 20% of sporadic cases and in up to 80% of hereditary cases.[2]

Paragangliomas are benign neoplasms in most cases; overall, less than 10% of all paragangliomas have been cited to be malignant.[2] In the head and neck, malignancy seems to be more common in vagal paragangliomas (16% to 19%) when compared with carotid body tumors (6%) and jugulartympanic tumors (2% to 4%).[2] There are no accepted histopathological criteria for malignancy, although the diagnosis of a malignant paraglioma can only be made when there is metastasis to nonneuroendocrine tissue.[2] In head and neck paragangliomas, metastases are most frequently found in cervical lymph nodes; distant sites, which include lung, liver, bone and skin, are very rare.[2,14]

The clinical presentation of a paraganglioma varies based on the tumor location. Jugulartympanic paragangliomas (Fig. 1) present with pulsatile tinnitus (84%) and hearing loss (76%) and frequently cause dysfunction of the cranial nerves VII–XII with large tumors.[15,16] Tympanic (Fig. 2) and jugular paragangliomas often present to the otolaryngologist as a bluish, pulsating mass behind the eardrum.[17]

In contrast, carotid body paragangliomas (Fig. 3) present as a painless, slowly enlarging mass lateral to the tip of the hyoid bone.[14] On physical examination, the tumor typically reveals a rubbery, nontender mass along the anterior border of the sternocleidomastoid. The tumor is mobile from side to side, but limited vertically because of the tumor's attachment to the carotid artery (Fontaine sign).[14] A carotid bruit or pulsatile character of the tumor strengthens the diagnosis. Neurologic deficits of cranial nerves VII, IX, X, XI, and XII can be found in some cases.[14] A painless neck mass is also the most frequent symptom in patients with a vagal paraganglioma (Fig. 4).[18] The tumor most commonly arises from the inferior (nodose) ganglion; however, it can arise from any point along the course of the nerve. Miller and colleagues[18] described their experience with a group of 19 vagal paraganglioma patients. The most frequent presenting symptoms were the presence of a neck mass (n = 14) and hoarseness (n = 7), followed by pharyngeal fullness (n = 5), dysphagia (n = 4), dysphonia (n = 4), pain (n = 4), cough (n = 3), and aspiration (n = 1).

In order to establish a diagnosis of a head and neck paraganglioma, imaging is essential.[19] Depending on the location and extent of the tumor, the following imaging modalities are frequently used: B-mode ultrasonography in combination with color-coded Doppler ultrasonography, computed tomography (CT), MR imaging, and digital subtraction angiography.[19] The most common radioligand for imaging of paragangliomas is In 111-DTPA-D-Phe1-octreotide (Fig. 5).

The different treatment options for paragangliomas include surgical excision, endovascular embolization, conventional radiotherapy, and stereotactic radiosurgery.[20] In selected cases, a watchful approach with repeat imaging may be warranted.

This article discusses normal anatomy and imaging techniques, imaging protocols, imaging findings/pathology, diagnostic criteria, differential diagnosis, and pearls/pitfalls/variants as they relate to paragangliomas involving the skull base. Finally, a brief bulleted list is presented describing what the referring physician needs to know.

NORMAL ANATOMY AND IMAGING TECHNIQUE
Normal Anatomy

The 3 most common paragangliomas of the head and neck are the carotid body, jugular, and tympanic tumors.[5] These tumors are located in the following areas: the carotid body paraganglioma is located at the carotid bifurcation; the jugular paraganglioma is located at the jugular foramen/bulb; and the tympanic paraganglioma is located at the cochlear promontory.[21] Therefore, paragangliomas of the head and neck require extensive anatomic knowledge of the jugular foramen, middle ear, and anterolateral neck.

Jugular fossa (JF) anatomy is important for understanding glomus jugular and tympanic paraganglioma pathology and imaging. The JF is a deep depression located in the temporal bone and cradles the jugular bulb. The JF is located directly behind the entrance of the carotid canal, lateral to the anterior half of the occipital condyle, medial to the stylomastoid foramen, posteromedial to the styloid process, and posteroinferior to the middle ear cleft. The foramen can be divided into anteromedial as well as posterolateral compartments. The anteromedial compartment contains the glossopharyngeal nerve, inferior petrosal sinus, and meningeal branch of the ascending pharyngeal artery. The posterolateral compartment contains the vagus and spinal accessory nerves. Tympanic paragangliomas typically arise from the tympanic plexus formed by tympanic nerve (Jacobson nerve), a branch of the glossopharyngeal nerve. The plexus of nerves lies on the cochlear promontory of the middle

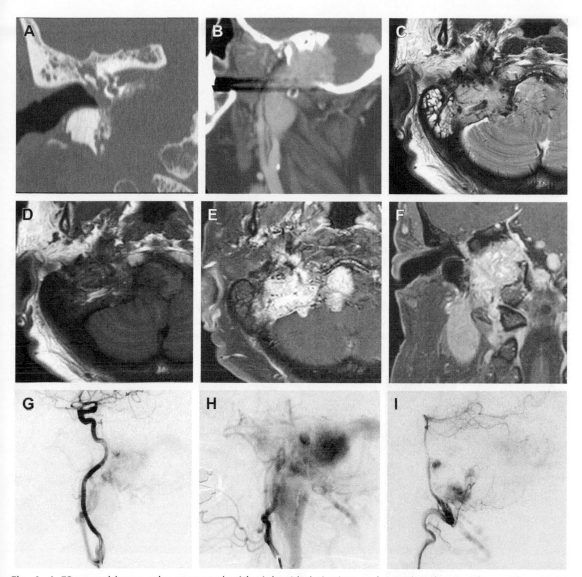

Fig. 1. A 52-year-old man who presented with right-sided tinnitus and complete hearing loss with a bluish pulsating mass behind the right tympanic membrane consistent with a jugular paraganglioma. (*A*) Coronal thin-section CT of the temporal bones shows a large mass expanding the jugular foramen extending into the middle ear cavity with erosion and a "moth-eaten" pattern of the jugular foramen, jugular plate. (*B*) Sagittal contrast-enhanced CT of the neck and skull base shows a large enhancing mass in the right jugular vein extending into the jugular foramen, middle ear, and bony labyrinth with intracranial extension. (*C–E*) Axial MR imaging T2-weighted image (*C*), T1-weighted image (*D*), and postcontrast fat-saturation T1-weighted image (*E*) at the level of the jugular foramen show a mass expanding the jugular foramen, which is hypointense on T1-weighted images, isointense/hyperintense on T2-weighted images, and enhances intensely after contrast injection. Signal voids related to the high flow in the tumor are common with a "salt-and-pepper appearance." The "pepper" component is caused by multiple areas of signal void, interspersed with the "salt" component, which is caused by hyperintense foci produced by slow flow or subacute hemorrhage on both T2- and T1-weighted images. (*F*) Coronal postcontrast fat-saturation T1-weighted image shows the full extent of the enhancing mass extending into the jugular vein, jugular foramen, middle ear cavity, bony labyrinth with intracranial extension. (*G–I*) Lateral right ICA (*G*), right ECA (*H*), and right VA (*I*) angiogram show a large hypervascular mass with arterial venous shunting centered within the jugular foramen extending inferior within the jugular vein and superior to the level of the internal auditory canal. The arterial supply is off of the enlarged muscular branches from the VA, the ascending pharyngeal artery, posterior auricular artery, occipital artery, and posterior inferior cerebellar artery.

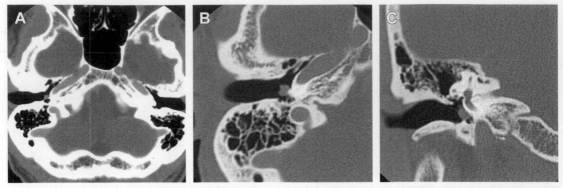

Fig. 2. A 41-year-old woman who presented with tinnitus and hearing loss consistent with a tympanic paraganglioma. (A) Axial contrast-enhanced CT of the temporal bones shows an enhancing mass in the right middle ear cavity. (B) Axial thin-section bone window CT scan of the temporal bones shows a soft tissue mass in the right middle ear cavity with no evidence of bone destruction. (C) Coronal thin-section bone window CT scan of the temporal bones again shows a soft tissue mass in the right middle ear cavity with no evidence of destruction of the JF.

ear. The inferior tympanic artery, which is a branch of the ascending pharyngeal artery, accompanies the nerve and usually also occupies a groove in the promontory.

Carotid body paragangliomas originate from the glomus body at the carotid bifurcation between the external carotid artery (ECA) and the internal carotid artery (ICA). Thus, it is important to

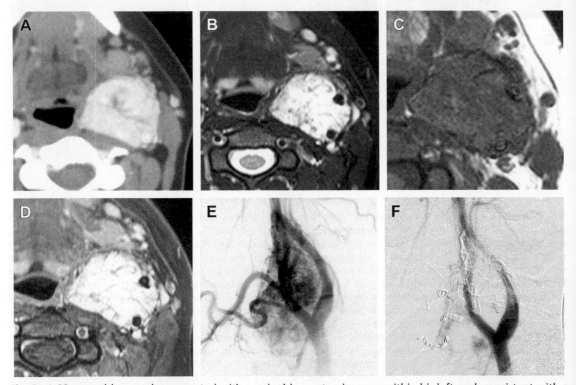

Fig. 3. A 32-year-old man who presented with a palpable nontender mass within his left neck consistent with a carotid body paraganglioma. (A) Axial contrast-enhanced CT of the neck shows a left-sided hypervascular mass splaying the internal and external carotid arteries. (B–D) Axial MR imaging T2-weighted image (B), T1-weighted image (C), and postcontrast fat-saturation T1-weighted image (D) show a hyperintense mass with flow voids splaying the carotid bifurcation on the T2-weighted image (B), which is isointense on T1-weighted image (C), and diffusely enhances after the administration of contrast. (E, F) Lateral left common carotid angiograms show a hypervascular mass with arterial venous shunting splaying the carotid bifurcation. Postembolization left common carotid angiogram (F) shows no filling of the hypervascular mass.

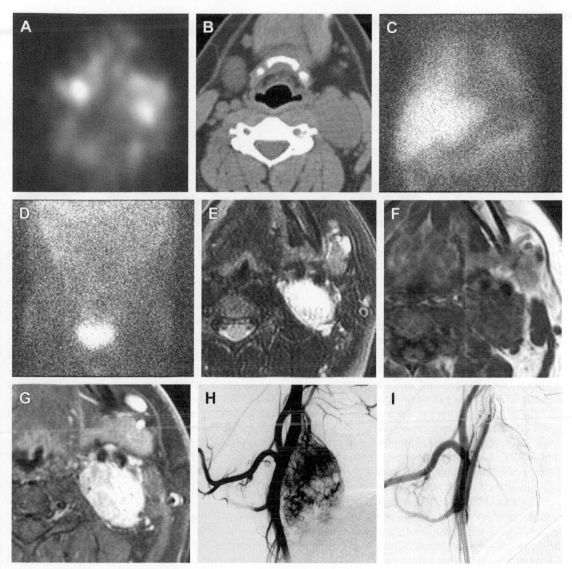

Fig. 4. A 25-year-old man with VHL syndrome who presented with a palpable nontender mass in his left neck with hoarseness consistent with a vagal paraganglioma. (A–D) Axial I-123 MIBG scan shows increased radiotracer uptake in the left neck (A), which corresponds to the mass seen on the unenhanced CT (B). The area in the right neck is normal uptake in the submandibular gland. I-123 MIBG coronal images over the chest (C) and abdomen (D) show no increase in radiotracer uptake. (E–G) Axial MR imaging T2-weighted image (E), T1-weighted image (F), and postcontrast fat-saturation T1-weighted image (G) show a hyperintense mass with flow voids without splaying of the carotid bifurcation on the T2-weighted image (E), which is isointense on the T1-weighted image (F), and diffusely enhances after the administration of contrast (G). (H, I) Lateral left common carotid angiogram (H) shows a hypervascular mass with arterial venous shunting displacing the ICA anterior. Postembolization left common carotid angiogram (I) shows no filling of the hypervascular mass.

understand the neurovascular relationship of the ICA as well as the ECA branches in the anterolateral neck. Nerves that pass between the ICA and ECA are at risk during surgery, including the glossopharyngeal nerve, superior laryngeal nerve (vagal branch), and pharyngeal nerve (vagal branch). However, with extension of the tumor, the hypoglossal nerve and the mandibular nerve (facial branch) may also be involved.

Imaging Technique

Along with medical history and targeted physical examination, imaging plays an important role in the diagnosis and management of head and neck paragangliomas. Initial imaging is usually done with CT and/or MR imaging.[22] Angiography is usually performed after the diagnosis is established for preoperative assessment. Functional

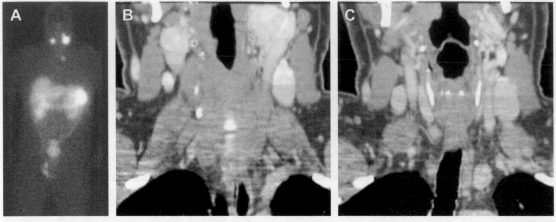

Fig. 5. A 29-year-old woman who presented with bilateral palpable nontender neck masses. This case shows the value of In-111 octeotide in demonstrating sites of multiple disease. (*A*) Coronal total body In-111 octreotide scan shows increased radiotracer uptake bilateral in the neck and in the left upper mediastinum. (*B, C*) Corresponding coronal contrast-enhanced CT images show the enhancing tumors within the neck (*B*) and (*C*) within the left upper mediastinum.

imaging with nuclear medicine radiotracers is used to evaluate for multifocal disease or distant metastases, but is not standard practice.

The initial imaging modality of choice to assess temporal bone involvement and to visualize bony structures and tumor extension is a high-resolution CT (HRCT) scan (<1 mm) in the axial, direct tumor plane, and reconstructed coronal plane.[23] However, when a suspicious mass is identified on a noncontrast HRCT, a contrast-enhanced temporal bone CT can help differentiate an intensely enhancing paraganglioma from other benign and malignant tumors of the skull base.[24] Compared with HRCT, multiplanar MR imaging with T1- and T2-weighted images along with gadolinium-enhanced images provides superior soft tissue details and identification of intracranial tumor extension.[22–24]

The imaging modality of choice for preoperative planning and tumor characterization is angiography. Angiography can identify the highly vascular tumor and provide important preoperative vascular mapping before surgical excision, and when indicated, embolization of the dominant arterial feeders can be performed before tumor resection.[23,25] Furthermore, angiography can characterize collateral vessels that must be spared during surgery and can provide further information about the patency of the venous system and multifocal nature of the tumor.[23]

Staging of the tumor for multifocal or distant metastases is done with nuclear medicine imaging and is becoming more sensitive and specific, but is not standard practice yet. The most common radioligand is In 111-DTPA-D-Phe1-octreotide, which has been shown to be superior to I-131 and I-123 metaiodobenzylguanidine (MIBG) in

clinical trials.[26–28] However, novel radiotracer F-18 FDOPA (fluorodopa) PET/CT is highly sensitive (>95%) and specific (95%–100%) for head and neck paraganglioma detection, but is not readily available at most sites.[29–33] Rapidly emerging radiotracer Ga-68 SSTa (Ga-68-labeled somatostatin analogues) combined with PET/CT could evolve as the new imaging standard of reference for imaging of paragangliomas and does not require a cyclotron to make the tracer.[34–38]

Imaging Protocols

CT and MR imaging protocols for imaging jugular, tympanic, and carotid body paragangliomas are included in **Tables 1–6**.

At the authors' institution, a biplane neck and cerebral angiogram is performed before surgical resection. The bilateral common carotid, internal carotid, external carotid, and vertebral arteries (VAs) are selectively catheterized with a 4-French vertebral catheter.

Nuclear medicine imaging is performed with I-123 MIBG and (In 111-DTPA-D-Phe1)-octreotide. When MIBG is radiolabeled with I-123, up to 10 mCi/m² can be administered. After intravenous administration, there is rapid uptake of MIBG mainly in the liver, and in lesser amounts in the lungs, heart, and salivary glands. A limited number of patients may show activity in normal adrenals, lung, skeletal, muscle, and blocked thyroid glands. Although the uptake in normal adrenal glands is very low, hyperplastic adrenals and tumors such as pheochromocytoma, neuroblastoma, and other tumors with neurosecretory granules have a relatively higher uptake. Significant clearance of

Table 1
Computed tomographic protocol of skull base: evaluation of a jugular paraganglioma

		HD750	VCT
Please position the patient's head so the Hard Palate is perpendicular to the table top.			
1. SUPINE SCOUTS: AP and LATERAL			
2. SUPINE AXIAL SCAN: START below skull base, END above petrous ridges			
Average CTDIvol = 65	Scan Type	Helical	Helical
NV CTDIvol = 65	HiRes Mode	On	n/a
Average CTDIvol = 84	Gantry Rot Time / Length	0.8s Full	0.8s Full
NV CTDIvol = 84	Detector Coverage	20 mm	20 mm
	Slice Thickness	0.625 mm	0.625 mm
	Interval	0.625 mm	0.625 mm
	Pitch	0.531:1	0.531:1
100cc ISOVUE 300 @ 2cc/s	Speed	10.62	10.62
	KVP	140	140
	mA	200	160
	ASIR % (SS or VS)	VS30	SS30
	% of Dose reduction	None	20 (mA x 0.8)
	Recon Mode	Plus IQ Enh	Plus IQ Enh
	DFOV	18-20	18-20
	SFOV	Head	Head
	Algorithm	HD Standard	Standard
	WW / WL	90 / 35	90 / 35
	Delay (if contrast ordered)	45s	45s
	RECON 2:		
	Slice Thickness	0.625 mm	0.625 mm
	Interval	0.625 mm	0.625 mm
	DFOV	18-20	18-20
	ASIR % (SS or VS)	VS30	SS30
	Recon Mode	Plus IQ Enh	Plus IQ Enh
	Algorithm	HD Bone Plus	Bone Plus
	WW / WL	4000 / 1000	4000 / 1000
3. MPRs: Axial & Coronal & Sagittal reformats in both Standard and Bone algorithm			
	Thickness	1.25 mm	1.25 mm
	Spacing	1.25 mm	1.25 mm
	DFOV	Optimize	Optimize
	Render Mode	Average	Average
	WW/WL (Bone)	4000 / 1000	4000 / 1000
	WW/WL (Standard)	90 / 35	90 / 35

Abbreviations: HD750, GE HD750 CT scanner; VCT, GE VCT 64 slice CT scanner.

I-123 MIBG from the liver and the spleen occurs within 72 hours. I-123 MIBG—In adrenal medullary tumors, initial images may be obtained 2 to 3 hours after injection. Images may also be obtained at 18 to 24 hours, and as late as 48 hours after injection. Most pheochromocytomas are visualized at 24 hours. However, because of the short half-life of I-123 MIBG, images may not be possible at times when background (eg, liver) activity is low and imaging would be optimal. Small amounts of radioactivity are used in diagnosis; radiation received is low and considered safe. Single-photon emission computed tomography (SPECT) is feasible with I-123 MIBG.

Ten micrograms of the octreotide can also be labeled to 3 mCi of In-111 (I-123 has also been

Table 2
Computed tomographic protocol of temporal bones: evaluation of a tympanic paraganglioma

		HD750	VCT

A BB marker MUST BE placed on the patient's right cheek regardless of the patients position during the scanning.
Please position the patient's head so the Hard Palate is perpendicular to the table top

1. SUPINE SCOUTS: AP and LATERAL
2. SUPINE AXIAL SCAN: START below mastoid process, END above petrous ridge apex, INCLUDE entire mastoid, IAC, & EAC

			HD750	VCT
Average CTDIvol =	73	Scan Type	Helical	Helical
NV CTDIvol =	73	HiRes Mode	On	n/a
Average CTDIvol =	93	Gantry Rot Time / Length	0.6s Full	0.6s Full
NV CTDIvol =	93	Detector Coverage	20 mm	20 mm
		Slice Thickness	0.625 mm	0.625 mm
100cc ISOVUE 300 @ 2cc/s		Interval	0.312 mm	0.312 mm
		Pitch	0.531:1	0.531:1
		Speed	10.62	10.62
		KVP	140	140
		mA	295	240
		ASIR % (SS or VS)	VS40	SS30
		% of Dose reduction	None	20 (mA x 0.8)
		Recon Mode	Plus	Plus IQ Enh
		SFOV	Head	Head
		DFOV	9.6	9.6
		Algorithm	Bone Plus	Bone Plus
		WW / WL	3200 / 400	3200 / 400
		Delay (If contrast ordered)	45s	45sec

RECON 1: for right side, RAZ coordinates ~R35
RECON 2: for left side, RAZ coordinates ~L35
RECON 3: for entire head

	HD750	VCT
Algorithm	HD Standard	Standard
DFOV	18	18
Slice Thickness	1.25 mm	1.25 mm
# of Images/Rotation	1.25 mm	1.25 mm
ASIR % (SS or VS)	SS40	SS30
Recon Mode	Plus IQ Enh.	Plus IQ Enh
WW / WL	90 / 35	90 / 35

3. MPRs: Coronal & Sagittal reformats in HD Bone algorithm of both Right and Left side separate

	HD750	VCT
DFOV	Optimize	Optimize
Thickness	0.625 mm	0.625 mm
Spacing	0.312 mm	0.312 mm
Render Mode	Average	Average
WW/WL (HD Bone)	3200 / 400	3200 / 400

4. RETROS: IF CONTRAST IS ORDERED, Do axial recons of both right and left side in a HD STANDARD algo @ 9.6 DFOV
Then do Coronal & Sagittal MPRs in HD Standard of both right and left

used). The dose of In-111 should be increased to 6 mCi if SPECT imaging is to be performed. SPECT imaging may increase the sensitivity of the examination and give better anatomic delineation compared with planar views.[39] The agent must be used within 6 hours of preparation. Images are obtained at 4 hours (over the area of interest) and 24 hours (from the head to the midthigh level) following injection. The examination is positive in 80% to 90% of cases by 4 hours. Planar images are obtained with a double-head or large field-of-view gamma camera, equipped with medium-energy, parallel hole collimators. The pulse height analyzer windows are centered over both In-111 photopeaks (172 keV and 245 keV) with a window

width of 20%. The acquisition parameters for planar images are 300,000 preset counts or 15-minute view of the head and neck and 500,000 counts or 15 minutes for the remainder of the body. Generally, 5- to 10-minute images are required for the images. A whole-body examination may be performed using a scan speed of 3 cm/min. Using higher scan speeds, such as 8 cm/min, will result in failure to recognize small lesions or lesions with a low density of somatostatin receptors.[39] For SPECT images with a triple-headed camera, the acquisition parameters are 40 steps or 3° each, 64 × 64 matrix, and at least 30 seconds per step (45 seconds for brain SPECT). Delayed images at 48 hours may also be obtained if

Table 3
Computed tomographic protocol of the neck: evaluation of a carotid body tumor

Have the patient remove dental work if possible.
Please mark all palpable masses with a BB marker.
Please position the patient's head so the Hard Palate is perpendicular to the table top.
1. SCOUTS: AP and Lateral
2. AXIAL SCAN: START mid orbit, END below clavicular heads (No gantry angle)
    ** If patient Hx includes "Vocal Cord Paralysis", please make sure to END scan through the Aortic Arch **
    Please center the scan group to include skin to skin anatomy of the head & neck structures

		Scan Type	Helical	Helical
Average CTDIvol =	16			
NV CTDIvol =	29	HiRes Mode	Off	n/a
Average CTDIvol =	18	Gantry Rot Time / Length	0.8s Full	0.8s Full
NV CTDIvol =	29	Detector Coverage	20 mm	20 mm
		Slice Thickness	1.25 mm	1.25 mm
		Interval	1.25 mm	1.25 mm
125 mls ISOVUE 300 @ 2ml/s		Speed	19.37	19.37
Split bolus injection		Pitch	0.969:1	0.969:1
2 injections (50 & 75 mls)		KVP BMI < 30	100	100
separated by a 2 minute		KVP BMI ≥ 30.1	120	120
delay.		Auto mA (min/max)	100 / 450	100 / 450
		Noise Index / Smart mA	30.36/ Off	26.4 / Off
		% of Dose reduction	30 (NI x 1.2)	30 (NI x 1.2)
Start the injector &		ASIR % (SS or VS)	SS60	SS60
the scanner together.		Recon Mode	Plus IQ Enh	Plus IQ Enh
		DFOV	20 - 24	20 - 24
Please instruct patient		SFOV	Small Body	Small Body
to **NOT** swallow during		Algorithm	Standard	Standard
the scan.		WW / WL	450 / 75	450 / 75
		Delay	180s	180s

DIRECT MPRs are turned on to auto batch the Standard Algo Series, **Coronal & Sagittal**
2 mm q 2 mm in all the rooms.

RECON 2

	HD750	VCT
Slice Thickness	1.25 mm	1.25 mm
Interval	1.25 mm	1.25 mm
DFOV	20 - 24	20 - 24
ASIR % (SS or VS)	SS60	SS60
Recon Mode	Plus IQ Enh	Plus IQ Enh
Algorithm	Bone Plus	Bone Plus
WW / WL	4000 / 1000	4000 / 1000

***If Neck is ordered with CAP or Chest CT, please scan the CAP or Chest CT
first and then scan the neck with a 35 second delay. Make sure to have the patient
set up in the coronal head holder, so you minimize the time between the two scans.....
then all you need to do between the exams is, bring the patient's arms to their sides, scout for
the neck, and set up the neck scan. This should take only 2 minutes.***

necessary—particularly if there is a large amount of bowel activity on 24-hour images (a laxative should also be used to help clear bowel activity).[39]

PATHOLOGY/IMAGING FINDINGS
Pathology

Jugulartympanic and carotid body paragangliomas manifest as a well-defined lobulated solid mass. The mass has a fibrous pseudocapsule exterior with interior cut surface containing multiple blood vessels.[40,41] Cellular architecture consists of chief cells and sustentacular cells that are surrounded by fibromuscular stroma.[41,42] The biphasic cellular architecture allows for

identification of S-100 and chromogranin structural proteins with immunohistochemical techniques to identify the tumor.[42,43]

Imaging Findings

Jugulartympanic paragangliomas
CT and MR imaging are the first-line imaging modalities in the localization and delineation of these tumors. CT of the temporal bone optimizes visualization of bone erosion.[23] Jugular paragangliomas are centered on the jugular foramen and can involve the hypotympanum. Early in the disease process, the JF is enlarged with irregular margins. With growth of the tumor, disease progression produces a typical "moth-eaten" pattern of the

Table 4
MR imaging protocol for jugular paraganglioma: cranial nerve V protocol

Examination Code MR70553	Series Description	Sag T1 TSE	AX DWI	AX T1 FLAIR	AX T2 STAR	AX T2 TSE
Patient	Patient position	Supine	Supine	Supine	Supine	Supine
Position	Patient orientation	Head first	Head first	Head first	Head first	Head first
	Coil type	Base/HN	Base/HN	Base/HN	Base/head	Base/HN
	Slice orientation	Sagittal	Axial	Axial	Axial	Axial
Coverage	—	Whole brain	Whole brain & CN V	Whole brain	Whole brain	Top of frontal sinus to C3 including mandible
Geometry	Field of view	230	256	254 × 200	254 × 200	160
	Voxel size	FH 0.78 AP 0.78	RL 1.5 AP 1.5	AP 0.69 RL 0.94	AP 0.9 RL 1.12	AP 0.60 RL 0.60
	Slice thickness	5/1	5/1	5/1	5/1	4/1
	Sense factor	1.6	4	1.5	1.8	2
	No. slices	21	25	25	25	34
	Fold-over direction	AP	AP	RL	RL	RL
Contrast	Scan mode	MS	MS	MS	MS	MS
	Technique	IR	SE	IR	FFE	SE
	Fast imaging mode	TSE	EPI	TSE	—	TSE
	TSE factor	5	SS	27	—	15
	TE	10	Shortest	125	In-phase 16.11	80
	TR	Shortest	Shortest	11,000	Shortest	Shortest
	Flip angle	—	90	—	18	90
	Fat saturation	—	SPIR	SPIR	—	—
Motion	NSA	1	2	1	1	2
Scan time	Scan duration	3:42	2:45	2:45	1:19	2:21

T1 MAP 30/15/05	AX T1 Perfusion	+/− AX T1 FLAIR	+AX e-T-HRIVE	+COR e-THRIVE	+AX T1 SE
Supine	Supine	Supine	Supine	Supine	Supine
Head first	Head first	Head first	Head first	Head first	Head first
Base/HN	Base/HN	Base/HN	Base/HN	Base/HN	Base/HN
Axial	Axial	Axial	Axial	COR	Axial
Cover ROI (tumor)	Cover ROI (tumor)	Top of frontal sinus to C3 including mandible	Top of frontal sinus to C3 including mandible	Frontal sinus to posterior pons	Whole brain
200 × 240	200 × 240	160	180	180	254 × 201
RL 1	RL 1	AP 0.6	AP 0.80	AP 0.8	AP 0.9
AP 1	AP 1	RL 0.75	RL 0.79	RL 0.79	RL 1.14
2.5/–	2.5/–	4/	0.60/–	0.6/–	5/1
2/1	2/1	1.6	2	1.5	—
48	48	34	250	200	25
AP	AP	RL	RL	RL	RL
3D	3D	MS	3D	3D	MS
FFE	FFE	IR	FFE	FFE	SE
—	—	TSE	TFE	TFE	—
—	—	7	SS	SS	—
Shortest	Shortest	20	Shortest	Shortest	10
Shortest	Shortest	2000	Shortest	Shortest	500–800
30/15/05	30	—	10	10	90
—	—	—	SPAIR	SPAIR	—
4	4	1	3	3	1
:53/:35/:35	5:33	4:12	5:03	5:03	2:55

Contrast Agent: Multihance.
Adult contrast dosage: 0.2 mL/kg body weight (ie, $^{3}/_{4}$ adult dose for routine brains and spines).
Method of administration: Intravenous butterfly injection.

Table 5
MR imaging protocol for evaluation of a tympanic paraganglioma: internal auditory canal/cranial nerve VII (IAC/CNVIII)

Examination Code MR70553	Series Description	SAG T1	AX DWI	AX T2 FLAIR	AX T2 STAR	AX 3D Drive	AX T2 THIN	+/− AX T1 THIN	+COR T1 THIN	+AX T1
Patient	Patient position	Supine	Supine	Supine	Supine	Supine	Supine	Supine	Supine	Supine
Position	Patient orientation	Head first	Head first	Head first	Head first	Head first	Head first	Head first	Head first	Head first
	Coil type	Base/head	Base/head	Base/head	Base/head	Base/head	Base/head	Base/head	Base/head	Base/head
	Slice orientation	Sagittal	Axial	Axial	Axial	Axial	Axial	Axial	Coronal	Axial
Coverage	—	Whole brain	Whole brain	Whole brain	Whole brain	Cover IACs	Cover IACs	Cover IACs	Cover IACs	Whole brain
Geometry	Field of view	240 × 240	256 × 256	230 × 185	254 × 200	160 × 160	180 × 180	180 × 180	180 × 180	230 × 185
	Voxel size	FH 0.78	RL 1.5	AP 0.69	AP 0.9	AP 0.55	AP 0.74	AP 0.74	FH 0.8	AP 1.89
		AP 0.78	AP 1.5	RL 0.94	RL 1.12	RL 0.55	RL 0.74	RL 0.92	RL 0.94	RL 1.14
	Slice thickness/gap	5	4	5	5/1	0.55	2	2	2.5	1
	Sense factor	1.6	4	1.5	1.8	1.5	1.6	—	—	—
	No. slices	21	28	25	25	50	18	18	15	25
	Fold-over direction	AP	AP	RL	RL	RL	RL	RL	RL	R/L
	—									
Contrast	Scan mode	MS	MS	MS	MS	3D	MS	MS	MS	MS
	Technique	IR	SE	IR	FFE	SE	SE	SE	SE	SE
	Fast imaging mode	TSE	EPI	TSE	—	TSE	TSE	—	—	—
	TSE factor	5	—	27	—	40	22	—	—	—
	TE	10	Shortest	125	In-phase 16	Shortest	90	8	10.5	10
	TR	Shortest	Shortest	11,000	Shortest	1500	3000	500	550–750	500–800
	Flip angle	—	90	—	18	90	90	90	90	90
	Fat saturation	—	SPIR	SPIR	—	—	—	—	—	—
Motion	NSA	1	2	1	1	1	1	1	1	1
Scan time	Scan duration	4:48	1:22	2:45	1:18	5:28	2:06	4:06	3:31	2:48

Contrast Agent: Multihance.
Adult contrast dosage: 0.2 mL/kg body weight (ie, ³⁄₄ adult dose for routine brains and spines).
Method of administration: Intravenous butterfly injection.
Notes: Reformat 3D drive in both SAG and COR planes separately for left and right IAC.

Table 6
MR imaging protocol for evaluation of a carotid body or vagal paraganglioma

Examination Code MR70543	Series Description	AX DWI	AX T2 FLAIR	SAG T1 TSE	AX DWI NECK	AX T2 F/S THIN	+/− AX T1 mDIXON THIN	*AX DYN e-THRIVE	+AX T1 SE
Patient	Patient position	Supine	Supine	Supine	Supine	Supine	Supine	Supine	Supine
Position	Patient orientation	Head first	Head first	Head first	Head first	Head first	Head first	Head first	Head first
	Coil type	Base/HN	Base/HN	Base/HN	Base/HN	Base/HN	Base/HN	Base/HN	Base/HN
	Slice orientation	Axial	Axial	Sagittal	Axial	Axial	Axial	Axial	Axial
Coverage	—	Whole brain	Whole brain	Whole neck	Whole neck	Hard palate to thor. inlet	Hard palate to thor. inlet	Hard palate to hyoid bone	Whole brain
Geometry	Field of view	256	230 × 185	240	256	200 × 220	200 × 220	260	254 × 201
	Voxel size	RL 1.5 AP 1.5	AP 0.69 RL 0.94	FH 0.8 AP 0.8	RL 1.5 AP 1.5	RL 0.95 FH 0.95	RL 0.95 FH 0.95	RL 1.016 AP 1.45	AP 0.9 RL 1.14
	Slice thickness/ gap	4/1	5/1	4/1	4/1	4/1	4/1	4/1	5/1
	Sense factor	3	1.7	2	4	2	1.6	2	—
	No. slices	35	25	34	28	40	40	26	25
	Fold-over direction	AP	RL	AP	AP	AP	AP	AP	RL
Contrast	Scan mode	MS	MS	MS	MS	MS	MS	MS	MS
	Technique	SE	IR	SE	SE	SE	IR	FFE	SE
	Fast imaging mode	EPI	TSE	TSE	EPI	TSE	TSE	—	—
	TSE factor	SS	27	5	SS	24	5	—	—
	TE	Shortest	125	10	Shortest	120	Shortest	Shortest	10
	TR	Shortest	11,000	400–650	Shortest	—	400–650	Shortest	500–800
	Flip angle	90	90	90	90	90	90	70	90
	Fat saturation	SPIR	SPIR	—	SPIR	SPAIR	—	SPIR	—
Motion	NSA	1	1	1	1	3	2	1	1
Scan time	Scan duration	1:26	2:45	4:26	1:26	3:56	4:53	2:34/30 s	2:55

Contrast Agent: Multihance.

Adult contrast dosage: 20 mL multihance.

Method of administration: Intravenous 10-s delay power injection @ 2 mL/s.

Notes: First scan is the prescan with a manual pause. Begin scan and injection at the same time.
Adult 3T Philips Ingenia 08/25/2014 DA.

jugular foramen.[44–46] The pattern represents erosion of the jugular foramen, jugular plate, or surrounding bony labyrinth.[23] Careful attention must be given to the relationship between the tumor and the bony covering on the jugular bulb (the jugular plate). Erosion of the jugular plate suggests a jugular paraganglioma. With contrast administration, the tumor has marked intratumoral vessel enhancement.[23,47]

MR imaging helps evaluate intracranial extension and soft tissue destruction. The tumor will spread toward the area of least resistance most commonly into the middle ear cleft and within the jugular vein.[48] However, with disease progression, the tumor can also spread to involve the petrous carotid canal, Eustachian tube, and carotid sheath, and extend intracranially.[48,49] Similar to carotid body paragangliomas, the tumor appears hypointense on T1-weighted images, isointense/hyperintense on T2-weighted images, and enhances intensely after gadolinium injection on MR imaging.[23,47] Signal voids related to the high flow in the tumor are common with a "salt-and-pepper appearance."[50,51] The "pepper" component is caused by multiple areas of signal void, interspersed with the "salt" component, which is caused by hyperintense foci produced by slow flow or subacute hemorrhage on both long TR and short TR images.[7] Diffusion-weighted imaging may be helpful for preoperative characterization and assessment of prognosis; however, further research needs to be performed to determine its role.[52]

Carotid body paraganglioma

B-mode sonography in combination with color-coded Doppler sonography is an inexpensive, noninvasive, readily available diagnostic tool that can be useful for imaging cervical paragangliomas. For this article, the authors concentrate on the cross-sectional CT and MR imaging findings of the respective tumors. CT of a carotid body paraganglioma shows a mass arising from carotid bifurcation with splaying of the carotid bifurcation; the ECA is displaced anteriorly, and both the ICA and internal jugular vein are displaced posteriorly.[19,53] After contrast administration, the tumor will show rapid enhancement.[23,47] MR imaging can provide further soft tissue characterization with the tumor appearing hypointense/isointense on T1-weighted images and hyperintense on T2-weighted images, and enhancing with gadolinium.[23,47]

Preoperative Imaging

Angiography

Angiography serves multiple purposes. First, it provides complementary diagnostic information by showing the characteristic, highly vascular nature of these tumors. Second, it allows for identification of dominant feeding vessels that can be embolized to reduce blood loss before surgical resection. Third, it identifies collateral vessels from the carotid artery and VAs that must be spared during surgery. Fourth, contralateral venous system patency can be assessed and major venous sinus occlusion from the tumor can be confirmed. Fifth, it can identify multifocal tumors.

The typical findings of a paraganglioma seen on angiography are a homogenous vascular tumor blush, enlarged feeding arteries supplying the tumor, the presence of arteriovenous shunts, and dilated venous outflow vessels.[54,55] Carotid body tumors show a vascular mass arising from carotid bifurcation with splaying of the carotid bifurcation (lyre sign), the ECA displaced anteriorly, and both the ICA and internal jugular vein displaced posteriorly.[56] The most common feeding artery is the ascending pharyngeal artery (branch of the ECA).[55,57] However, the ICA, ECA, and posterior circulation branches as well as contralateral arteries should be examined for arterial feeding vessels. Embolization is suggested for jugular and carotid body paragangliomas; however, given their small size and easy accessibility, embolization of tympanic paragangliomas is not usually performed.

Embolization

The goal of tumor embolization is to selectively occlude the ECA feeders using intratumoral deposition of the embolic material.[58] The embolic agents commonly used include the following: polyvinyl alcohol, trisacryl microspheres, liquid n-butyl cyanoacrylate (n-BCA; Trufill; Cordis Neurovascular Inc, Miami Lakes, FL, USA), ethyl vinyl alcohol copolymer (EVOH; Onyx; ev3, Irvine, CA, USA), gelfoam pledgets, and microcoils.

The embolization is ideally performed from 24 to 72 hours before the surgical resection to allow time for maximal thrombosis of the occluded vessels and prevent recanalization of the occluded arteries or formation of collateral arterial channels.[59,60] Preoperative embolization is cost-effective and tends to shorten operative time by reducing blood loss and the period of recovery.[61]

Treatment begins by first obtaining a detailed cerebral angiogram that includes selective injections of the common carotid artery, ICA, ECA, VA, and thyrocervical and costocervical trunks of the subclavian artery. A microcatheter is then advanced using fluoroscopic guidance into the artery supplying the tumor, and a microcatheter angiogram is performed to check for dangerous anastomoses between the ECA and ICA or VAs.

The appropriate embolic agent is then injected using constant fluoroscopic monitoring, making sure to avoid reflux of embolic material and being vigilant for any dangerous anastomoses. If critical anastomoses are present, the anastomotic connection can be occluded using coils, and then the particulate embolization can be performed. Ideally, the embolic material is deposited at the arteriolar/capillary level. If there is arteriovenous shunting within the tumor, the particle size may need to be increased to prevent passage into the venous side. Proximal occlusion of the arterial feeders is inadequate because it allows arterial collateralization and may make surgical removal more difficult.

The authors prefer using trisacryl microspheres of 100 to 300 microns because these particles allow more distal penetration into the tumor bed and better devascularization.[62] However, one should always be aware of the possible risk for devascularizing the cranial nerves (the vasa nervosum are usually smaller than 60 microns) and the skin. In addition to potential central and peripheral nervous system damage, undesired embolization of normal external carotid territories can cause mucosal and tongue necrosis, laryngeal damage, and ocular damage. Smaller particles may also increase the risk for tumoral hemorrhage and swelling.[63] When embolizing the arterial pedicles that might also supply the cranial nerves (eg, the stylomastoid branch of the occipital artery (OA) or the neuromeningeal trunk of the ascending pharyngeal artery (APA)), the authors increase the particle size to from 300 to 500 microns. Similarly, the authors generally avoid liquid embolic agents (eg, n-BCA or EVOH), preferring to use a transarterial approach with particulate material, because liquid embolic agents can potentially occlude the arterial supply to the cranial nerves and may pass through the tiny anastomoses into the intracranial circulation.

Direct percutaneous puncture of tumors using fluoroscopic, ultrasound, or CT guidance has also been described as a method to embolize several different tumors. The method was initially reported for use in tumors in which conventional transarterial embolization was technically impossible because of the small size of the arterial feeders or involvement of branches arising from the ICA or VA feeding the tumor.[64] Examples include large tumors with supply from the ICA, VA, or ophthalmic artery for which devascularization from an intra-arterial approach using a microcatheter may not be possible or for which there may be significant risk for reflux of particles into the intracranial circulation or the retina. Excellent results obtained using this technique have extended its application to smaller and less complex tumors.[65] Direct and easy access to the vascular tumor bed that is not hampered by arterial tortuosity, the small size of the arterial feeders, atherosclerotic disease, or catheter-induced vasospasm is the main advantage of this technique.[66–68]

Complete devascularization of the tumor can be obtained with decreased risk to the patient by using direct tumoral injection of n-BCA or Onyx. n-BCA and Onyx are liquid embolic agents for presurgical embolization of cerebral arteriovenous malformations. Onyx is a nonadhesive liquid embolic agent that is supplied in ready-to-use vials in a mixture with EVOH, dimethyl sulfoxide solvent (DMSO), and tantalum. Currently 6% (Onyx 18) and 8% (Onyx 34) EVOH concentrations (dissolved in DMSO) are available in the United States. Onyx is mechanically occlusive but nonadherent to the vessel wall. Its nonadherent properties allow for a slow single injection of the embolic agent over a long period of time. During direct injection, if unfavorable filling of the normal vascular structures occurs, the injection can be stopped and resumed after 30 seconds to 2 minutes. Solidification will occur in the embolized portion of the tumor. The injection can then be restarted, with Onyx taking the path of least resistance and filling another portion of the tumor. As the result of its properties, Onyx may potentially allow for a more controlled injection with better penetration into the tumor bed compared with n-BCA. Another benefit is that it advances in a single column, thus reducing the risk for involuntary venous migration. The authors have recently shown a decrease in blood loss during surgical resection of hypervascular tumors treated with direct injection of Onyx when compared with particulate embolization.[69,70]

The authors perform percutaneous injection of n-BCA or Onyx by placing an 18-gauge, or 20-gauge needle into the tumor using fluoroscopic, ultrasound, or CT guidance. After the needle is correctly located within the vascular bed of the tumor, a constant reflux of blood is observed. Contrast agent is injected through the needle and a tumor angiogram is obtained to assess for arterial reflux, venous drainage, potential for extravasation, and to determine which vascular compartment of the tumor will be filled with n-BCA or Onyx. The injection of the embolic agent is then performed using negative roadmap. The procedure is stopped after complete devascularization is achieved, as determined by nonvisualization of intratumoral flow, or if the risk for potential arterial reflux into the intracranial circulation is considered to be high.

Table 7
Fisch criteria for jugulartympanic paragangliomas

Class	Location and Extension of Paraganglioma
A	Paragangliomas that arise along tympanic plexus on promontory
B	Paragangliomas with invasion of hypotympanon; cortical bone over jugular bulb intact
C1	Paragangliomas with erosion of carotid foramen
C2	Paragangliomas with destruction of carotid canal
C3	Paragangliomas with invasion of carotid canal; foramen lacerum intact
C4	Paragangliomas invading foramen lacerum and cavernous sinus
De1/2	Paragangliomas with intracranial extension, no infiltration of interarachnoidal space; De1–De2 according to displacement of dura (De1 = <2 cm, De2 = >2 cm)
Di1/2/3	Paragangliomas with intracranial and intradural extension; Di1–Di3 according to depth of invasion into posterior fossa (Di1 = <2 cm, Di2 = between 2 and 4 cm, Di3 = >4 cm)

DIAGNOSTIC CRITERIA

Several diagnostic criteria have been purposed for carotid body and jugulartympanic paragangliomas, although none have gained universal acceptance. The most common criteria for jugulartympanic paragangliomas are the Fisch and Glasscock/Jackson criteria (**Tables 7 and 8**).[71–73] The most common criteria for carotid body paragangliomas are classified according to the Shamblin criteria (**Table 9**).[74] These different classifications help to describe the anatomic location as well as the spread of the tumor, helping to guide surgical management.[75] A newer trend of classifying paragangliomas genetically is also emerging because of the 30% prevalence of germline mutations in head and neck paragangliomas.[9,76] Thus, genetic counseling should be offered for all head and neck paragangliomas.[9,76]

DIFFERENTIAL DIAGNOSIS

The most common clinical presentation of jugular-tympanic paraganglioma is pulsatile tinnitus, hearing loss, and a pulsatile mass. According to a review of 8 previously published articles, the causes of pulsatile tinnitus are represented in **Table 10** for 620 patients.[17,77–83] The 4 most common causes were venous anatomic variants/abnormalities (27%), arterial stenosis (16%), indirect arteriovenous fistulas (7%), and vessel-rich tumors (7%).[17,77–83] Paragangliomas are classified within the category of vessel-rich tumors. The main imaging differential diagnosis for a jugular-tympanics paraganglioma includes metastases, meningioma, hemangiomas, Paget disease, melanoma, middle ear adenoma, acoustic neuroma (rarely pulsatile), and an endolymphatic sac tumor.[84–86] The main imaging differential for a carotid body paraganglioma includes a vagal

Table 8
Glasscock/Jackson criteria for jugulartympanic paragangliomas

Glomus Tympanicum	
I	Small mass limited to promontory
II	Tumor completely filling middle ear space
III	Tumor filling middle ear and extending into mastoid
IV	Tumor filling middle ear, extending into the mastoid or through tympanic membrane to fill the external auditory canal; may extend anterior to carotid

Glomus Jugulare	
I	Small tumor involving jugular bulb, middle ear, and mastoid
II	Tumor extending under internal auditory canal; may have intracranial canal extension
III	Tumor extending into petrous apex; may have intracranial canal extension
IV	Tumor extending beyond petrous apex into clivus or infratemporal fossa; may have intracranial canal extension

Table 9
Shamblin criteria for carotid body paragangliomas

Group	Relation to Carotid Artery and Resectability
I	Includes small tumors that are only loosely adherent to the adventitia of the artery and are easily removed
II	Tumors are somewhat larger and are more densely adherent to the artery and even infiltrate the vessel wall; sharp adventitial dissection is required for their removal
III	Includes very large tumors that encircle or encompass the artery to such an extent that a portion of the vessel must be resected for complete removal of the tumor with subsequent grafting

schwannoma, vagal neurofibroma, a lymph node mass, glomus vagale paraganglioma (same abnormality but located more rostrally), and aneurysms of the carotid artery.

PEARLS, PITFALLS, VARIANTS

- CT is useful when bony erosion occurs; a "moth-eaten" pattern is typical.
- On MR imaging, paragangliomas may show a "salt-and-pepper" appearance with the "salt" being blood products from hemorrhage and the "pepper" being flow voids due to high vascularity.
- Erosion of the jugular plate suggests a jugular paraganglioma.
- Carotid body tumors on imaging show a vascular mass arising from carotid bifurcation with splaying of the carotid bifurcation (lyre sign).

Table 10
Causes of pulsatile tinnitus

Cause	Percentage
Arterial	**21**
Stenosis	16
Aneurysm	2
Anatomic variants	3
Venous	**31**
Intracranial hypertension	4
Anatomic variants/abnormalities	27
Arteriovenous transition	**20**
Indirect arteriovenous fistulas	7
Direct arteriovenous fistulas	2
Arteriovenous malformations	0
Vessel-rich tumors	7
Capillary hyperemia	3
Other	**8**
Unknown	**20**

- Important to rule out an aberrant ICA as a vascular mass behind the tympanic membrane. Vagal paraganglioma usually displaced the ICA anterior.

WHAT THE REFERRING PHYSICIAN NEEDS TO KNOW

- At least 30% of patients with a paraganglioma and no other risk factor harbor a genetic mutation.
- All patients, including those with a sporadic tumor, should be referred for a genetic consultation.
- The most common paraganglioma locations of the head and neck in descending order are the carotid body, jugular, tympanic, and vagal paragangliomas.
- Classic tumor syndromes associated with a high incidence of paragangliomas include MEN II, VHL disease, and NF I.
- Jugulartympanic paragangliomas present with pulsatile tinnitus and hearing loss and frequently cause dysfunction of the cranial nerves VII–XII with large tumors.
- CT and MR imaging with contrast are the primary imaging modalities for evaluation of a paraganglioma.
- In 111-DTPA-D-Phe1-octreotide is the preferred radiotracer to evaluate for multiple paragangliomas.
- Carotid body and vagal paragangliomas present as a painless, slowly enlarging mass in the neck.
- The different treatment options for paragangliomas include embolization, surgical excision, conventional radiotherapy, watchful waiting, and stereotactic radiosurgery.

SUMMARY

The most common paraganglioma locations of the head and neck are the carotid body, jugular, tympanic, and vagal paragangliomas. Syndromes associated with a high incidence of paragangliomas include MEN II, VHL disease, and NF I. All patients, including those with a sporadic tumor, should be referred for a genetic consultation. Jugular and tympanic paragangliomas commonly present with tinnitus and hearing loss, whereas carotid body and vagal paragangliomas usually present with nonpainful palpable neck mass. CT and MR imaging are the main modalities used for imaging diagnosis with angiography reserved for embolization and preoperative planning before surgical resection. Nuclear imaging with In-111 octreotide is useful in demonstrating sites of multiple disease. The different treatment options for paragangliomas include surgical excision, endovascular embolization, conventional radiotherapy, and stereotactic radiosurgery.

REFERENCES

1. Zak FG. An expanded concept of tumors of glomic tissue. N Y State J Med 1954;54(8):1153–65.
2. Lee JH, Barich F, Karnell LH, et al. National Cancer Data Base report on malignant paragangliomas of the head and neck. Cancer 2002;94(3):730–7.
3. Baysal BE. Hereditary paraganglioma targets diverse paraganglia. J Med Genet 2002;39(9):617–22.
4. Petropoulos AE, Luetje CM, Camarata PJ, et al. Genetic analysis in the diagnosis of familial paragangliomas. Laryngoscope 2000;110(7):1225–9.
5. Semaan MT, Megerian CA. Current assessment and management of glomus tumors. Curr Opin Otolaryngol Head Neck Surg 2008;16(5):420–6.
6. O'Leary MJ, Shelton C, Giddings NA, et al. Glomus tympanicum tumors: a clinical perspective. Laryngoscope 1991;101(10):1038–43.
7. Vogl T, Bisdas S. Differential diagnosis of jugular foramen lesions. Skull Base 2009;19(1):3–16.
8. Bacca A, Sellari Franceschini S, Carrara D, et al. Sporadic or familial head neck paragangliomas enrolled in a single center: clinical presentation and genotype/phenotype correlations. Head Neck 2013;35(1):23–7.
9. Boedeker CC, Neumann HP, Offergeld C, et al. Clinical features of paraganglioma syndromes. Skull Base 2009;19(1):17–25.
10. Favier J, Gimenez-Roqueplo AP. Genetics of paragangliomas and pheochromocytomas. Med Sci 2012;28(6–7):625–32.
11. Martins R, Bugalho MJ. Paragangliomas/pheochromocytomas: clinically oriented genetic testing. Int J Endocrinol 2014;2014:794187.
12. Lefebvre M, Foulkes WD. Pheochromocytoma and paraganglioma syndromes: genetics and management updates. Curr Oncol 2014;21(1):e8–17.
13. Neumann HP, Bausch B, McWhinney SR, et al. Germ-line mutations in nonsyndromic pheochromocytoma. N Engl J Med 2002;346(19):1459–66.
14. Patetsios P, Gable DR, Garrett WV, et al. Management of carotid body paragangliomas and review of a 30-year experience. Ann Vasc Surg 2002;16(3):331–8.
15. Fayad JN, Keles B, Brackmann DE. Jugular foramen tumors: clinical characteristics and treatment outcomes. Otol Neurotol 2010;31(2):299–305.
16. Offergeld C, Brase C, Yaremchuk S, et al. Head and neck paragangliomas: clinical and molecular genetic classification. Clinics (Sao Paulo) 2012;67(1):19–28.
17. Hofmann E, Behr R, Neumann-Haefelin T, et al. Pulsatile tinnitus-imaging and differential diagnosis. Dtsch Arztebl Int 2013;110(26):451–8.
18. Miller RB, Boon MS, Atkins JP, et al. Vagal paraganglioma: the Jefferson experience. Otolaryngol Head Neck Surg 2000;122(4):482–7.
19. Stoeckli SJ, Schuknecht B, Alkadhi H, et al. Evaluation of paragangliomas presenting as a cervical mass on color-coded Doppler sonography. Laryngoscope 2002;112(1):143–6.
20. Foote RL, Pollock BE, Gorman DA, et al. Glomus jugulare tumor: tumor control and complications after stereotactic radiosurgery. Head Neck 2002;24(4):332–8 [discussion: 338–9].
21. Taieb D, Varoquaux A, Chen CC, et al. Current and future trends in the anatomical and functional imaging of head and neck paragangliomas. Semin Nucl Med 2013;43(6):462–73.
22. Johnson MH. Head and neck vascular anatomy. Neuroimaging Clin N Am 1998;8(1):119–41.
23. Corrales CE, Fischbein N, Jackler RK. Imaging innovations in temporal bone disorders. Otolaryngol Clin North Am 2015;48(2):263–80.
24. Subedi N, Prestwich R, Chowdhury F, et al. Neuroendocrine tumours of the head and neck: anatomical, functional and molecular imaging and contemporary management. Cancer Imaging 2013;13(3):407–22.
25. Wanna GB, Sweeney AD, Haynes DS, et al. Contemporary management of jugular paragangliomas. Otolaryngol Clin North Am 2015;48(2):331–41.
26. Koopmans KP, Jager PL, Kema IP, et al. 111In-octreotide is superior to 123I-metaiodobenzylguanidine for scintigraphic detection of head and neck paragangliomas. J Nucl Med 2008;49(8):1232–7.
27. Le Rest C, Bomanji JB, Costa DC, et al. Functional imaging of malignant paragangliomas and carcinoid tumours. Eur J Nucl Med 2001;28(4):478–82.
28. Muros MA, Llamas-Elvira JM, Rodríguez A, et al. 111In-pentetreotide scintigraphy is superior to 123I-MIBG scintigraphy in the diagnosis and location of chemodectoma. Nucl Med Commun 1998;19(8):735–42.
29. Charrier N, Deveze A, Fakhry N, et al. Comparison of [111In]pentetreotide-SPECT and [18F]FDOPA-PET

in the localization of extra-adrenal paragangliomas: the case for a patient-tailored use of nuclear imaging modalities. Clin Endocrinol (Oxf) 2011;74(1):21–9.

30. Gabriel S, Blanchet EM, Sebag F, et al. Functional characterization of nonmetastatic paraganglioma and pheochromocytoma by 18F-FDOPA PET: focus on missed lesions. Clin Endocrinol (Oxf) 2013; 79(2):170–7.

31. King KSCC, Alexopoulos DK, Whatley MA, et al. Functional imaging of SDHx-related head and neck paragangliomas: comparison of 18F-fluorodihydroxyphenylalanine, 18F-fluorodopamine, 18F-fluoro-2-deoxy-D-glucose PET, 123I-metaiodobenzylguanidine scintigraphy, and 111In-pentetreotide scintigraphy. J Clin Endocrinol Metab 2011;96(9):2779–85.

32. Miederer M, Fottner C, Rossmann H, et al. High incidence of extraadrenal paraganglioma in families with SDHx syndromes detected by functional imaging with [18F]fluorodihydroxyphenylalanine PET. Eur J Nucl Med Mol Imaging 2013;40(6):889–96.

33. Timmers HJ, Chen CC, Carrasquillo JA, et al. Comparison of 18F-fluoro-L-DOPA, 18F-fluoro-deoxyglucose, and 18F-fluorodopamine PET and 123I-MIBG scintigraphy in the localization of pheochromocytoma and paraganglioma. J Clin Endocrinol Metab 2009;94(12):4757–67.

34. Janssen I, Blanchet EM, Adams K, et al. Superiority of [68Ga]-DOTATATE PET/CT to other functional imaging modalities in the localization of SDHB associated metastatic pheochromocytoma and paraganglioma. Clin Cancer Res 2015;21(17):3888–95.

35. Hofman MS, Lau WF, Hicks RJ. Somatostatin receptor imaging with 68Ga DOTATATE PET/CT: clinical utility, normal patterns, pearls, and pitfalls in interpretation. Radiographics 2015;35(2):500–16.

36. Kroiss A, Putzer D, Frech A, et al. A retrospective comparison between 68Ga-DOTA-TOC PET/CT and 18F-DOPA PET/CT in patients with extra-adrenal paraganglioma. Eur J Nucl Med Mol Imaging 2013; 40(12):1800–8.

37. Sharma P, Thakar A, Suman KC, et al. 68Ga-DOTA-NOC PET/CT for baseline evaluation of patients with head and neck paraganglioma. J Nucl Med 2013; 54(6):841–7.

38. Maurice JB, Troke R, Win Z, et al. A comparison of the performance of 68Ga-DOTATATE PET/CT and 123I-MIBG SPECT in the diagnosis and follow-up of phaeochromocytoma and paraganglioma. Eur J Nucl Med Mol Imaging 2012;39(8):1266–70.

39. Kwekkeboom D, Krenning EP, de Jong M. Peptide receptor imaging and therapy. J Nucl Med 2000; 41(10):1704–13.

40. Lack EE, Cubilla AL, Woodruff JM. Paragangliomas of the head and neck region: a pathologic study of tumors from 71 patients. Hum Pathol 1979;10(2):191–218.

41. Lack EE. Tumors of the adrenal gland and extra-adrenal paraganglioma. In: Rosai J, editor. Atlas of tumor pathology, series 3, fasc 19. Washington, DC: Armed Forces Institute of Pathology; 1997. p. 303–409.

42. Kliewer KE, Cochran AJ. A review of the histology, ultrastructure, immunohistology, and molecular biology of extra-adrenal paragangliomas. Arch Pathol Lab Med 1989;113(11):1209–18.

43. Kliewer KE, Wen DR, Cancilla PA, et al. Paragangliomas: assessment of prognosis by histologic, immunohistochemical, and ultrastructural techniques. Hum Pathol 1989;20:29–39.

44. Rao AB, Koeller KK, Adair CF. Paragangliomas of the head and neck: radiologic-pathologic correlation. Radiographics 1999;19(6):1605–32.

45. Lo WW, Solti-Bohman LG, Lambert PR. High-resolution CT in the evaluation of glomus tumors of the temporal bone. Radiology 1984;150(3):737–42.

46. Som PM, Reede DL, Bergeron RT, et al. Computed tomography of glomus tympanicum tumors. J Comput Assist Tomogr 1983;7(1):14–7.

47. Lee KY, Oh YW, Noh HJ, et al. Extraadrenal paragangliomas of the body: imaging features. AJR Am J Roentgenol 2006;187(2):492–504.

48. Sanna M, Piazza P, Shin S, et al. Microsurgery of skull base paragangliomas. Stuttgart (Germany): Thieme; 2013.

49. Phelps PD, Stansbie JM. Glomus jugulare or tympanicum? The role of CT and MR imaging with gadolinium DTPA. J Laryngol Otol 1988;102(9):766–76.

50. Olson WL, Dillon WP, Kelly WM, et al. MR imaging of paragangliomas. AJR Am J Roentgenol 1987; 148(1):201–4.

51. Vogl TJ, Juergens M, Balzer JO, et al. Glomus tumors of the skull base: combined use of MR angiography and spin-echo imaging. Radiology 1994; 192(1):103–10.

52. Aschenbach R, Basche S, Vogl TJ, et al. Diffusion-weighted imaging and ADC mapping of head-and-neck paragangliomas: initial experience. Klin Neuroradiol 2009;19(3):215–9.

53. Som PM, Sacher M, Stollman AL, et al. Common tumors of the parapharyngeal space: refined imaging diagnosis. Radiology 1988;169(1):81–5.

54. Wilson MA, Hillman TA, Wiggins RH, et al. Jugular foramen schwannomas: diagnosis, management, and outcomes. Laryngoscope 2005;115(8):1486–92.

55. Ramina R, Maniglia JJ, Fernandes YB, et al. Tumors of the jugular foramen: diagnosis and management. Neurosurgery 2005;57(1):59–68.

56. Muhm M, Polterauer P, Gstottner W, et al. Diagnostic and therapeutic approaches to carotid body tumors. Review of 24 patients. Arch Surg 1997;132(3):279–84.

57. Christie A, Teasdale E. A comparative review of multidetector CT angiography and MRI in the diagnosis of jugular foramen lesions. Clin Radiol 2010;65(3): 213–7.

58. Valavanis A, Christoforidis G. Applications of interventional neuroradiology in the head and neck. Semin Roentgenol 2000;35(1):72–83.

59. Kai Y, Hamada J, Morioka M, et al. Appropriate interval between embolization and surgery in patients with meningioma. AJNR Am J Neuroradiol 2002; 23(1):139–42.

60. Chun JY, McDermott MW, Lamborn KR, et al. Delayed surgical resection reduces intraoperative blood loss for embolized meningiomas. Neurosurgery 2002;50(6):1231–5 [discussion: 1235–7].

61. Dean BL, Flom RA, Wallace RC, et al. Efficacy of endovascular treatment of meningiomas: evaluation with matched samples. AJNR Am J Neuroradiol 1994;15(9):1675–80.

62. Wakhloo AK, Juengling FD, Van Velthoven V, et al. Extended preoperative polyvinyl alcohol microembolization of intracranial meningiomas: assessment of two embolization techniques. AJNR Am J Neuroradiol 1993;14(3):571–82.

63. Kallmes DF, Evans AJ, Kaptain GJ, et al. Hemorrhagic complications in embolization of a meningioma: case report and review of the literature. Neuroradiology 1997;39(12):877–80.

64. Quadros RS, Gallas S, Delcourt C, et al. Preoperative embolization of a cervicodorsal paraganglioma by direct percutaneous injection of onyx and endovascular delivery of particles. AJNR Am J Neuroradiol 2006;27(9):1907–9.

65. Abud DG, Mounayer C, Benndorf G, et al. Intratumoral injection of cyanoacrylate glue in head and neck paragangliomas. AJNR Am J Neuroradiol 2004;25(9):1457–62.

66. Gemmete JJ, Chaudhary N, Pandey A, et al. Usefulness of percutaneously injected ethylene-vinyl alcohol copolymer in conjunction with standard endovascular embolization techniques for preoperative devascularization of hypervascular head and neck tumors: technique, initial experience, and correlation with surgical observations. AJNR Am J Neuroradiol 2010;31(5):961–6.

67. Gemmete JJ, Patel S, Pandey AS, et al. Preliminary experience with the percutaneous embolization of juvenile angiofibromas using only ethylene-vinyl alcohol copolymer (Onyx) for preoperative devascularization prior to surgical resection. AJNR Am J Neuroradiol 2012;33(9):1669–75.

68. Shah HM, Gemmete JJ, Chaudhary N, et al. Preliminary experience with the percutaneous embolization of paragangliomas at the carotid bifurcation using only ethylene vinyl alcohol copolymer (EVOH) Onyx. J Neurointerv Surg 2012;4(2):125–9.

69. Gao M, Gemmete JJ, Chaudhary N, et al. A comparison of particulate and onyx embolization in preoperative devascularization of juvenile nasopharyngeal angiofibromas. Neuroradiology 2013;55(9):1089–96.

70. Griauzde J, Gemmete JJ, Chaudhary N, et al. A comparison of particulate and Onyx embolization in preoperative devascularization of carotid body tumors. Neuroradiology 2013;55(9):1113–8.

71. Jackson CG, Glasscock ME, Harris PF. Glomus tumors. Diagnosis, classification, and management of large lesions. Arch Otolaryngol 1982;108(7):401–10.

72. Fisch U, Pillsbury HC. Infratemporal fossa approach to lesions in the temporal bone and base of the skull. Arch Otolaryngol 1979;105(2):99–107.

73. Oldring D, Fisch U. Glomus tumors of the temporal region: surgical therapy. Am J Otol 1979;1(1):7–18.

74. Shamblin WR, ReMine WH, Sheps SG, et al. Harrison EG carotid body tumor (chemodectoma). Clinicopathologic analysis of ninety cases. Am J Surg 1971;122(6):732–9.

75. Sanna M, Jain Y, De Donato G, et al. Management of jugular paragangliomas: the Gruppo Otologico experience. Otol Neurotol 2004;25(5):797–804.

76. Papathomas TG, de Krijger RR, Tischler AS. Paragangliomas: update on differential diagnostic considerations, composite tumors, and recent genetic developments. Semin Diagn Pathol 2013;30(3):207–23.

77. Dietz RR, Davis WL, Harnsberger HR, et al. MR imaging and MR angiography in the evaluation of pulsatile tinnitus. AJNR Am J Neuroradiol 1994;15(5):879–89.

78. Herraiz C, Aparicio JM. Diagnostic clues in pulsatile tinnitus. Acta Otorrinolaringol Esp 2007;58(9):426–33.

79. Mattox DE, Hudgins P. Algorithm for evaluation of pulsatile tinnitus. Acta Otolaryngol 2008;128(4): 427–31.

80. Sismanis A. Pulsatile tinnitus. Otolaryngol Clin North Am 2003;36(2):389–402.

81. Sonmez G, Basekim CC, Öztürk E, et al. Imaging of pulsatile tinnitus: a review of 74 patients. Clin Imaging 2007;31(2):102–8.

82. Waldvogel D, Mattle HP, Sturzenegger M, et al. Pulsatile tinnitus—a review of 84 patients. J Neurol 1998;245(3):137–42.

83. Base SC, Kim DK, Yeo SW, et al. Single-center 10-year experience in treating patients with vascular tinnitus: diagnostic approaches and treatment outcomes. Clin Exp Otorhinolaryngol 2015;8(1):7–12.

84. Weissman JL, Hirsch BE. Imaging of tinnitus: a review. Radiology 2000;16(2):342–9.

85. Hofmann E, Arps H, Schwager K. Paragangliomas of the head and neck region (glomus tumors). Radiologie uptodate 2009;9(4):339–53.

86. Gehrking E, Gliemroth J, Missler U, et al. Main symptom: "pulse-synchronous tinnitus". Laryngorhinootologie 2000;79(9):510–6.

Surgical Treatment of Tinnitus

David J. Eisenman, MD*, Taylor B. Teplitzky, BS

KEYWORDS

- Tinnitus • Surgery for tinnitus • Objective tinnitus • Sigmoid sinus wall anomalies

KEY POINTS

- Most patients with objective tinnitus, whether pulse-synchronous or not, will have an identifiable and frequently treatable cause.
- Venous etiologies of pulse-synchronous tinnitus are the most common.
- A thorough diagnostic evaluation must look for causes of abnormal sound production and abnormal sound perception.
- Vascular studies must include venous phases, with particular attention to imaging the transverse and sigmoid sinuses.
- Subtle sigmoid sinus wall anomalies will only be detected with high-resolution appropriately windowed computed tomography.

INTRODUCTION

Surgery for tinnitus can be divided into procedures directed specifically at elimination of tinnitus versus those directed at an independent primary otopathology whose symptoms include tinnitus (Table 1). For the latter, although there may be an independent primary goal for which the surgery is undertaken, tinnitus may be expected to improve secondarily. This article will address both tinnitus-specific and nontinnitus-specific procedures for objective and subjective causes.

Tinnitus is defined as the abnormal perception of sound in the absence of an external sound source. Objective tinnitus has traditionally referred to a sound that can be heard by another listener aside from the patient. This term can be misleading, since it is highly dependent on the degree of attention the examiner pays and the tools employed. However, if one defines objective tinnitus as that which, based on its auditory characteristics and other features, is thought to arise from an objective, mechanical sound source, the

ambiguity is eliminated. Objective tinnitus can be pulsatile (or, more precisely, pulse-synchronous) or nonpulsatile. Surgical intervention for tinnitus relief is most commonly performed for objective tinnitus.

Using the same rationale for definition, a so-called subjective tinnitus is that which, based on the presumed etiology and pathophysiology, is thought to be caused by a purely electrochemical phenomenon. This type of abnormal sound perception cannot be heard by an objective listener no matter the sensitivity of the listening equipment. Although commonly perceived as a continuous tone, it too can often have rhythmicity, such as that of chirping crickets, although it is only very rarely truly pulse-synchronous or regularly rhythmic. Throughout this article, sounds thought to arise from an objective, mechanical sound source will be referred to as objective tinnitus, and those arising from a purely electrochemical phenomenon will be referred to as subjective tinnitus.

The authors have nothing to disclose.
Department of Otorhinolaryngology—Head and Neck Surgery, University of Maryland School of Medicine, 16 South Eutaw Street, Suite 500, Baltimore, MD 21201, USA
* Corresponding author.
E-mail address: deisenman@smail.umaryland.edu

Neuroimag Clin N Am 26 (2016) 279–288
http://dx.doi.org/10.1016/j.nic.2015.12.010
1052-5149/16/$ – see front matter © 2016 Elsevier Inc. All rights reserved.

neuroimaging.theclinics.com

Table 1
Surgical options for tinnitus

Tinnitus Specific Surgery	Surgery with Secondary Benefit on Tinnitus
Subjective	Subjective
Vagus nerve stimulation	Hearing restoration surgery
Cochlear or cochlear nerve stimulation	Ossicular chain reconstruction
Deep brain stimulation	Cochlear implantation
Intratympanic steroid injection	Other implantable hearing devices (eg, bone
Objective	conduction devices)
Tensor tympani and/or stapedius	Intratympanic steroid Injection (eg, for Meniere's disease
tenotomy	or sudden sensorineural hearing loss)
Sigmoid sinus wall reconstruction	Objective
Eustachian tube dysfunction	Superior canal dehiscence syndrome
Middle ear ventilation	Excision of paraganglioma
Eustachian tuboplasty	
Internal jugular vein ligation	

CLINICAL EVALUATION

For a detailed discussion of the clinical evaluation of the patient with tinnitus, please refer to Hertzano R, Teplitzky TB, and Eisenman DJ: Clinical Evaluation of Tinnitus, in this issue. To summarize, the focus of the evaluation must be directed both at identifying potentially treatable causes and at assessing the impact of the tinnitus on the patient's daily activity and well-being. It is important to distinguish early on between objective and subjective causes, because the focus of the evaluation will differ significantly. A thorough history and complete head and neck examination are the critical foundation upon which the further evaluation rests. Complete audiometry will identify and classify any associated, and possibly causative, hearing loss. Most patients with subjective tinnitus have underlying hearing loss.[1] If the audiogram demonstrates symmetric sensorineural hearing loss, the tinnitus itself is perceived bilaterally or with no lateralization, and there are no other associated symptoms or physical examination findings of concern, then no further diagnostic evaluation is required.

The differential diagnosis for pulse-synchronous tinnitus should be divided into causes due to abnormal sound production (eg, transverse sinus stenosis, sigmoid sinus wall anomalies, acquired dural vascular lesions) and those due to abnormal sound perception (eg, third mobile window syndromes) (Table 2). There are also some causes whose pathophysiology is uncertain, such as migraine and Meniere's disease. If during the initial clinical assessment a particular category is found

Table 2
Differential diagnosis for pulsatile tinnitus

Abnormal Sound Perception	Abnormal Sound Production
Eustachian tube dysfunction	Carotid stenosis
Patulous eustachian tube	Durai arteriovenous malformation
Eustachian tube dysfunction with diminished middle ear	High riding carotid artery
aeration	Sigmoid sinus wall anomalies
Causes of conductive hearing loss	Sigmoid sinus wall dehiscence
External auditory canal obstruction	Sigmoid sinus diverticulum
External auditory canal stenosis	Transverse sinus stenosis
Middle ear disease	Paraganglioma
Tympanic membrane perforation	Glomus tympanicum
Ossicular discontinuity	Glomus jugulare
Otosclerosis	Unknown or uncertain cause
Third mobile window syndromes	Migraine
Superior semicircular canal dehiscence	Meniere disease
Cochlear–carotid fistula	
Enlarged vestibular aqueduct	

to be the likely cause for the tinnitus, the remainder of the evaluation will be directed more specifically toward evaluation of this etiology. It is important to note that a significant majority of patients with pulse-synchronous tinnitus will have an identifiable, and often treatable, cause.[2]

Patients with a conductive hearing loss on the puretone audiogram must undergo immittance testing. Conductive hearing loss can be associated both with middle ear abnormalities, such as ossicular discontinuity or fixation, and with third mobile window syndromes, such as superior semicircular canal dehiscence. However, whereas patients with the former will typically have absent acoustic reflexes, in third mobile window syndromes, the reflexes should be present. Additionally, patients with a third mobile window will often have symptoms of dizziness with observable nystagmus, evoked by application of positive and negative pressure to the sealed external auditory canal (the so-called fistula test). Vestibular evoked myogenic potentials (VEMP) can also be helpful in distinguishing conductive hearing loss caused by stapes fixation from that of a third mobile window syndrome. With otosclerosis and other causes of stapes fixation, the VEMP responses are typically absent, because the fixed stapes does not provide sufficient mechanical stimulus to vibrate the otolithic organs. With third mobile window syndromes, on the other hand, responses are typically present at abnormally low thresholds.[3]

Radiographic imaging may be indicated following the initial clinical evaluation. Patients with asymmetric sensorineural hearing loss, or chronic, unilateral subjective tinnitus even with symmetric hearing, should undergo diagnostic magnetic resonance before and after administration of gadolinium contrast to look for lesions along the auditory pathway from the labyrinth to the brainstem. Patients with subjective tinnitus associated with other neurologic symptoms, such as vertigo, disequilbrium, headache, or other cranial neuropathies, should be tested with a similar protocol.

Diagnostic imaging is always indicated for patients with objective tinnitus, although there is controversy about the optimal imaging strategy. For pulse-synchronous objective tinnitus, the authors employ a modified computed tomography (CT) angiography brain protocol, as described in the article on venous abnormalities leading to tinnitus in this issue. Briefly, the contrast injection is delayed slightly to ensure venous enhancement, and the images are acquired with bone windows to allow for identification of fine bony deficiencies. This protocol allows for identification of otic capsule dehiscences causing third mobile window

syndromes, sigmoid sinus wall anomalies including subtle dehiscences, soft tissue lesions in the middle ear, and lesions in the jugular foramen. Many indirect signs of acquired dural vascular lesions can be identified as well, such as asymmetrically increased arterial feeders or venous collaterals, transcalvarial channels, inner table scalloping and asymmetric venous attenuation.[4] Asymmetric early venous filling, however, may be missed because of the delayed injection. If this study does not demonstrate a cause for the pulsatile tinnitus, digital subtraction angiography (DSA) is considered. DSA is not recommended as the initial study of choice, because this will not diagnose common causes such as sigmoid sinus wall dehiscence, middle ear abnormalities, or third mobile window syndromes. If DSA is undertaken, it is important to include venous phase images to look for dural venous sinus stenosis and other venous etiologies.

Underlying causes of nonpulse-synchronous objective tinnitus due to presumed middle ear myoclonus are rarely identified with diagnostic imaging. However, most clinicians still feel imaging is indicated to exclude a lesion along the cranial nerve pathways supplying the tensor tympani and stapedius muscles, or those that mediate the afferent pathways of their reflex contraction. This is best done with contrast-enhanced magnetic resonance of the brain with attention to the internal auditory canals and skull base.[5]

NONSPECIFIC TREATMENTS (IE, TREATMENTS FOR OTHER INDICATIONS WITH SECONDARY TINNITUS BENEFIT)

Most patients with severe hearing loss, whether conductive or sensorineural, report an associated, nonrhythmic, subjective tinnitus that likely results from the sensory deafferentation. Consequently, many procedures directed at hearing improvement will secondarily result in an improvement in tinnitus. Most patients who are candidates for cochlear implantation for bilateral, unaidable sensorineural hearing loss also have associated tinnitus. Studies have shown that most of these patients will report an improvement in their tinnitus following implantation.[6,7] Similarly, preliminary data have suggested that patients with unilateral sensorineural hearing loss and tinnitus who undergo implantation of an osseointegrated bone-conduction device for their hearing loss will also report improvement in their subjective tinnitus.[8,9] Intratympanic perfusion of steroids has been employed for a variety of idiopathic otopathologies that are commonly associated with tinnitus, including Meniere's disease, sudden sensorineural hearing loss, and acute labyrinthitis, among other disorders. Studies have shown that many patients undergoing intratympanic perfusion for inner ear diseases associated with tinnitus, particularly patients with Meniere disease, will also report improvement in the associated tinnitus following the procedure.[10]

In addition to a nonrhythmic subjective tinnitus, many patients with conductive hearing loss or conductive hyperacusis will also experience pulse-synchronous tinnitus. Clinical experience suggests that procedures to improve hearing for the former will usually result in improvement in the pulse-synchronous tinnitus, although systematic studies are lacking. Similarly, many, if not most, patients with pulse-synchronous tinnitus associated with superior canal dehiscence syndrome will report improvement in that symptom when canal occlusion or resurfacing procedures are performed.[11,12] However, there are insufficient data to determine if pulse-synchronous tinnitus alone is an appropriate indication for canal dehiscence surgery.

Finally, surgery for excision of a middle ear or jugular foramen paraganglioma that is also associated with pulse-synchronous tinnitus would be expected to relieve the symptom if the primary lesion is successfully removed.

SURGERY FOR PRIMARY INDICATION OF TINNITUS
Subjective Tinnitus

Surgical options directed primarily and specifically at remediation of subjective tinnitus are limited. Various approaches have been tried, but none has been demonstrated to be sufficiently reliable or effective for long-term control. Both implantable[13] and transcutaneous[14,15] vagus nerve stimulators have been tried for elimination of subjective tinnitus in pilot studies. Variable benefits were seen, but long-term efficacy data are still lacking, and this approach has not yet been employed in standard clinical practice. Although not a surgical intervention per se, worth mentioning are the many studies that have looked at the potential benefits of repetitive transcranial magnetic stimulation (rTMS). Despite numerous different approaches and trials, a thorough meta-analysis of the literature to develop evidence-based guidelines for use concluded that there was, at best, Level C evidence for its use, suggesting possible efficacy.[16]

The observation that tinnitus suppression is often a secondary benefit accruing from deep brain stimulation for other indications such as Parkinson disease[17,18] has led investigators to consider this option as a primary intervention for subjective tinnitus, although results are still preliminary.[19]

Similarly, the observation that most patients who undergo cochlear implantation for profound hearing loss have subjective tinnitus and find relief from it when using the device has led investigators to consider cochlear implantation solely for tinnitus relief. Consideration for implantation has been given to patients without hearing loss sufficiently severe to warrant implantation and in patients with only unilateral hearing loss for whom cochlear implantation might otherwise not be indicated.[20,21] Results have been variable, and tinnitus relief is still not considered a primary indication for cochlear implantation. Newer studies have combined electrical stimulation along with normal sound perception in cochlear implant users.[22] This approach, coupled with new cochlear implants and surgical techniques that allow for hearing preservation in implantees, may pave the way for further trials investigating the utility of cochlear implantation as a primary treatment for subjective tinnitus.

A review of 5 prospective, randomized trials that employed intratympanic steroids for primary treatment of refractory, subjective tinnitus found that only 1 trial demonstrated benefit to this approach versus a control group.[23] This trial was directed at patients with a duration of symptoms of less than 3 months,[24] and may not be representative of the more common group of chronic tinnitus sufferers seen in clinical practice.

Objective Tinnitus

Surgical intervention for objective tinnitus is both more commonly performed and more effective than that for subjective tinnitus. An objective, rhythmic, but nonpulse-synchronous, tinnitus is usually caused by middle ear myoclonus. Palatal myoclonus must also be included in the differential diagnosis, and should be excluded before considering surgery. The tensor tympani muscle, the stapedius, or both, can be the cause. Definitive differentiation of the muscle causing the symptom is not possible preoperatively, although when the symptom develops following facial nerve infection, inflammation, or trauma, the stapedius muscle is more likely to be the cause. The stapedius muscle is also likely responsible when the tinnitus is evoked by facial movements or loud sounds.[25]

Middle ear exploration with lysis of the tendon of the affected muscle, or both if the causative muscle is undetermined, can be performed after more conservative measures have failed.[5] There are no definitive trials with high-quality evidence demonstrating conclusive results and management guidelines, but there are many anecdotal studies supporting surgery when conservative measures fail.[26]

Pulsatile tinnitus is a common symptom of Eustachian tube dysfunction. Alterations in middle ear pressure produce a conductive hearing loss, which results in abnormally heightened self-perception of vascular somatosounds. Choice of an appropriate treatment approach requires distinguishing between the more common dilatory dysfunction with resultant hypofunction and underaeration of the middle ear, typically caused by nasopharyngeal and paranasal sinus inflammatory disorders or chronic otitis media, on the one hand, and patulous Eustachian tube, which is commonly seen in patients with rapid weight loss, on the other.

When dilatory dysfunction persists despite appropriate medical therapy, surgery should be considered. Ventilation tube insertion is the simplest and most common surgical intervention. This does not restore normal function, but simply obviates the consequences, both symptomatic and physiologic, of decreased middle ear ventilation. Because ventilation tubes pose a risk of otitis media with water exposure, and repeated insertion of tubes may lead to tympanic membrane damage in some patients, other, more physiologic approaches to restoration of function have been tried, most recently with Eustachian tube dilation using paranasal sinus balloon catheters. Results are still preliminary and vary between studies, but there is room for guarded optimism that this can be an effective independent or adjunctive treatment modality for selected patients.[27] Care must be taken both with patient selection and technique. The cartilaginous portion of the Eustachian tube is the only portion that can be safely and effectively dilated. For this reason, a patient who has had a lifetime of chronic otitis media with no rhinitic or nasopharyngeal pathology, and who has chronically poor Eustachian tube function, is not a good candidate for such a procedure, because the site of pathology is likely on the middle ear side of the tube, if not along its entire length altogether.

Various procedures have been tried for medically refractory symptoms of an abnormally patulous Eustachian tube. A recent systematic review found that there is no high-quality evidence defining appropriate medical therapy or failure of such therapy, supporting one specific surgical option over another, or demonstrating objective success rates of any procedure. Procedures employed have included ventilation tube insertion, hamulotomy, and occlusion or partial occlusion of the nasopharyngeal Eustachian tube orifice via endoscopic ligation, injection of bulking agents, cauterization, insertion of shims or fat grafts, and other techniques.[27,28]

Ligation of the internal jugular vein has been proposed and attempted for chronic pulsatile tinnitus. Although precise indications have not been established, it is most commonly employed for tinnitus associated with a high and/or dehiscent jugular bulb. Results are inconsistent, with only small numbers reported, and long-term results are not well known.[29,30] In addition to the risk of failure, the procedure also carries a risk of causing intracranial hypertension from decreased venous outflow. Additionally, even recent studies have not looked for associated sigmoid sinus wall anomalies, despite the fact that most affected patients are young women and likely in the same population at risk for such abnormalities. This is particularly significant, both because nonobstructing options would be available for treatment of these patients, and because many of these patients are already at an increased risk of intracranial hypertension. In an unequivocally worded letter to the editor of the journal *Otology and Neurotology*, 3 experienced and prominent neurotologists strongly warned against any major vessel ligation purely for the purposes of alleviating pulsatile tinnitus.[31]

SIGMOID SINUS WALL ANOMALIES

Sigmoid sinus wall anomalies (SSWAs) comprise sigmoid sinus diverticulum and dehiscence[32] (Fig. 1). A definitive classification scheme is still lacking, and other descriptors, such as sigmoid sinus ectasia, may better describe certain radiographic sigmoid sinus anomalies that may be associated with pulse-synchronous tinnitus. SSWAs are the most common finding on CT scans performed for a diagnosis of pulse-synchronous tinnitus or in patients with that symptom.[2,33,34] They are uncommonly found on CT scans performed for reasons other than pulse-synchronous tinnitus.[34,35] Definitive diagnostic criteria have yet to be established, and subtle dehiscences, and even sometimes larger diverticula, can still not be overlooked.

The precise etiology of these anomalies is unknown, although various lines of evidence have suggested an association with idiopathic intracranial hypertension (IIH) in at least some affected patients. In a large series of consecutive patients undergoing surgery for pulse-synchronous tinnitus associated with SSWA, Harvey and colleagues[32] showed that most subjects were women with elevated body mass index, similar to the

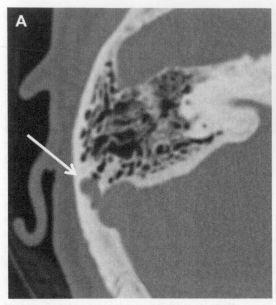
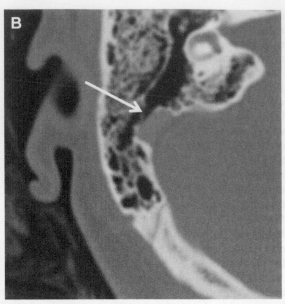

Fig. 1. Radiologic imaging demonstrating sigmoid sinus wall anomalies. (*A*) Arrow denotes right sigmoid sinus diverticulum. (*B*) Arrow indicating right sigmoid sinus dehiscence.

population affected by IIH. Similar findings were identified in a series from another center.[34] Comstock and colleagues[36] performed preoperative lumbar puncture under anesthesia in a small cohort of patients undergoing surgery for SSWA, and found an elevated mean opening pressure. Furthermore, Liu and colleagues[37] performed volumetric T1-weighted MRI on 33 subjects with unilateral pulse-synchronous tinnitus found to have an SSWA on high-resolution CT. They found a statistically elevated prevalence of numerous findings known to be associated with IIH in this cohort, such as empty sella, flattened posterior sclera, transverse sinus stenosis, optic nerve protrusion and/or tortuousity. and distension of the optic nerve sheath.

Clinical and radiographic evaluation of patients with suspected and confirmed SSWA has been described. All of the authors' patients with confirmed SSWA undergo formal neurophthalmologic evaluation to look for signs of IIH. Lumbar puncture is reserved for those with clinical findings warranting that procedure, as judged by the evaluating physician. Medical treatment of suspected or confirmed IIH should be undertaken before considering surgery. Specific radiographic findings that may be helpful to note for the referring physician are listed in **Box 1**.

Treatment of sigmoid sinus diverticulum via an endoluminal approach was first described in 3 independent case reports.[38–40] The first description of a transmastoid approach for repair of sigmoid sinus diverticulum was by Otto and

colleagues[41] in 2007. Sigmoid sinus dehiscence without diverticulum as a cause of pulse-synchronous tinnitus, and its successful repair via a transmastoid approach, was first described

---

Box 1
Sigmoid sinus wall anomalies: what a referring physician needs to know

- Presence of sigmoid sinus wall anomaly
  - Dehiscence and/or diverticulum
  - Unilateral or bilateral
  - Size
  - Location
- Presence of transverse sinus stenosis
  - Ipsilateral to symptoms
  - Contralateral to symptoms
  - Bilateral
  - Severity
- Dominance of transverse–sigmoid systems
  - Ipsilateral to symptoms
  - Contralateral to symptoms
  - Codominant
- Presence of empty sella
- Other signs of intracranial hypertension
- Exclusion of other causes of pulse-synchronous tinnitus

in 2011 in a surgical series of 13 consecutively treated patients.[42] Other series have since confirmed a high success rate of relief of pulse-synchronous tinnitus with transmastoid repair of SSWA.[32,36,43]

It is important for the radiologist to be familiar with the various techniques to be able to accurately interpret findings on postoperative imaging studies. Various techniques have been described for transtemporal procedures to treat pulsatile tinnitus caused by SSWA.[41,42,44] Otto and colleagues employed a variety of techniques in their small study, mostly free muscle or fascia grafts and bone wax to create a smooth sigmoid sinus surface. The same group has subsequently employed titanium miniplates affixed to the posterior ledge of the mastoid defect for extraluminal reduction of diverticula.[2] Guo and Wang have employed sigmoid sinus compression with cartilage, muscle, and fascia inserted deep to the posterior fossa bone overlying the sinus wall for ecstatic and markedly enlarged sigmoid sinuses, both with and without diverticula.[44]

Eisenman[42] described a standardized technique of sinus wall reconstruction for both diverticulum and dehiscence, referred to as sinus wall reconstruction. After exposure and decompression of the pathologic area via a transmastoid approach, the diverticulum, if present, is reduced with bipolar cautery. Bone is removed circumferential to the pathologic region until normal-appearing sigmoid sinus is decompressed, although this is not always possible with proximal lesions. If during the reduction bleeding is encountered, the affected area is covered with a thin layer surgical oxidized cellulose matrix. The sigmoid sinus is then covered with a layer of neural acellular dermal matrix or temporalis fascia, inserted deep to the petrous bone, superficial to the dura and sinus wall. The bony defect is then reconstructed with a layer of hydroxylapatite cement. This layer is then covered with a layer of autologous bone paté, over which the mastoid periosteal flap is tightly reapproximated. The layers of this reconstruction, and their relationship to the sigmoid sinus and overlying bone, are depicted in **Fig. 2**.

Postoperative imaging can be employed to check on the integrity of the reconstruction, its success in reducing a diverticulum or resurfacing a dehiscence, and to look for complications.

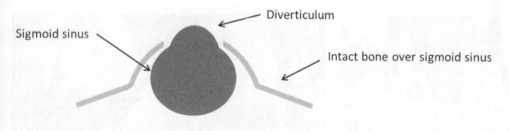

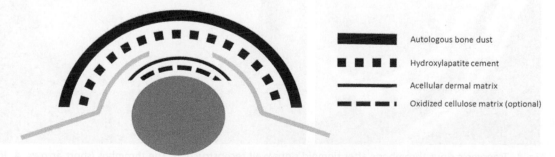

Fig. 2. Sinus wall reconstruction for sigmoid sinus wall anomalies. (A) Sigmoid sinus diverticulum before reconstruction demonstrating an area of dehiscent bone allowing an out-pouching of the sigmoid sinus through the defect. (B) Sigmoid sinus after surgical reconstruction of the dehiscent bone with 3 or 4 layers of material.

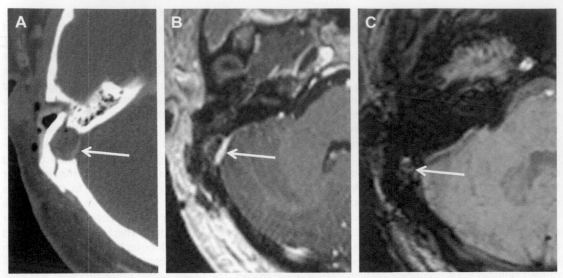

Fig. 3. Mass effect upon the sigmoid sinus by graft swelling after sinus wall reconstruction. (*A*) Marked compression of the sigmoid sinus lumen presumably from hypodense swollen graft material is evident. (*B*) Note that this appears as a filling defect confined to the surgical bed and does not propagate along the transverse sinus. (*C*) Lack of hypointensity on the Gradient Recalled Echo (GRE) image, indicating that this is not thrombosis.

The risk of symptomatic sigmoid sinus thrombosis (**Fig. 3**) is likely higher in this patient population than in patients undergoing transtemporal approaches for other pathologies. This may be because of the higher rate of associated preoperative transverse sinus stenosis in patients with SSWA, or because the procedure is more commonly performed on the dominant side.[32] The authors currently use a regimen of prophylactic perioperative anticoagulation to minimize this risk, although its efficacy is not yet proven. Postoperative thrombosis is treated with therapeutic anticoagulation. Measures to

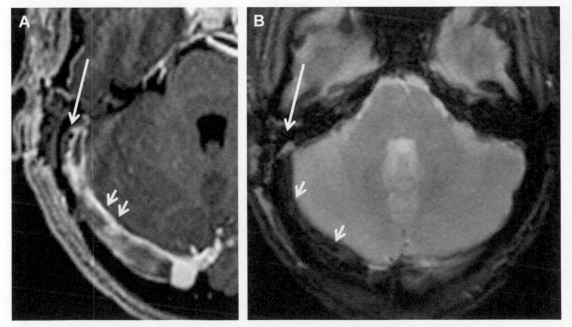

Fig. 4. Transverse sinus thrombosis after sigmoid sinus wall reconstruction. The thrombus (short *arrows*, *A*, *B*) is seen as a filling defect on the contrast enhanced T1W image (*A*) and is hypointense on the GRE image (*B*). The soft tissue graft (Surgicel and Alloderm) is the small nonenhancing filling defect indicated by the long arrows. Note that unlike thrombus, it is not hypointense on the GRE image.

decrease intracranial pressure acutely should be utilized as well if needed.

It is important to distinguish sigmoid sinus thrombosis from extraluminal compression (**Fig. 4**) on postoperative imaging. This can usually be accomplished with diagnostic MR Imaging and magnetic resonance angiography.[45] It is important to communicate with the surgeon to understand the surgical technique that was employed, and the anticipated layers of the reconstruction. Whereas the sigmoid sinus thrombosis may have a higher risk of propagation and is more likely to require anticoagulation, extraluminal compression, if asymptomatic, can usually be observed. For symptomatic extraluminal compression, consideration would need to be given to surgical re-exploration and revision, or angiography with angioplasty and/or stenting.

SUMMARY

Many surgical options exist for patients with chronic tinnitus. Subjective, nonrhythmic tinnitus is usually treated medically and behaviorally, although there are future possibilities for tinnitus-specific directed surgical intervention. The majority of cases of pulse-synchronous tinnitus will have an identifiable cause, many of which can be treated with surgical or angiographic interventions. Sigmoid sinus wall anomalies are a common cause of pulse-synchronous tinnitus. Different surgical approaches have been described, all with high rates of success. Radiologists must be familiar both with the subtleties of diagnosis and the expected postoperative imaging appearance to be able to work with the treating clinician in managing patients with these anomalies.

REFERENCES

1. Adams PF, Hendershot GE, Marano MA. Current estimates from the national health interview survey, 1996. Vital Health Stat 1999;200:1–203. Series 10, Data from the National Health Survey.
2. Mattox DE, Hudgins P. Algorithm for evaluation of pulsatile tinnitus. Acta Otolaryngol 2008;128(4): 427–31.
3. Merchant SN, Rosowski JJ. Conductive hearing loss caused by third-window lesions of the inner ear. Otol Neurotol 2008;29(3):282.
4. Narvid J, Do HM, Blevins NH, et al. CT angiography as a screening tool for dural arteriovenous fistula in patients with pulsatile tinnitus: feasibility and test characteristics. AJNR Am J Neuroradiol 2011; 32(3):446–53.
5. Park SN, Bae SC, Lee GH, et al. Clinical characteristics and therapeutic response of objective tinnitus due to middle ear myoclonus: a large case series. Laryngoscope 2013;123(10):2516–20.
6. Ruckenstein MJ, Hedgepeth C, Rafter KO, et al. Tinnitus suppression in patients with cochlear implants. Otol Neurotol 2001;22(2):200–4.
7. Souliere CR, Kileny PR, Zwolan TA, et al. Tinnitus suppression following cochlear implantation: a multifactorial investigation. Arch Otolaryngol Head Neck Surg 1992;118(12):1291–7.
8. Indeyeva YA, Diaz A, Imbrey T, et al. Tinnitus management with percutaneous osseointegrated auditory implants for unilateral sensorineural hearing loss. Am J Otolaryngol 2015;36(6):810–3.
9. Holgers KM, Håkansson BE. Sound stimulation via bone conduction for tinnitus relief: a pilot study: estimulación sonora por vía ósea para mejorar el acúfeno: un estudio piloto. Int J Audiol 2002; 41(5):293–300.
10. Garduño-Anaya MA, Couthino De Toledo H, Hinojosa-González R, et al. Dexamethasone inner ear perfusion by intratympanic injection in unilateral meniere's disease: a two-year prospective, placebo-controlled, double-blind, randomized trial. Otolaryngol Head Neck Surg 2005;133(2):285–94.
11. Teixido Michael, Seymour PF, Kung B, et al. Transmastoid middle fossa craniotomy repair of superior semicircular canal dehiscence using a soft tissue graft. Otol Neurotol 2011;32(5):877–81.
12. Beyea JA, Agrawal SK, Parnes LS. Transmastoid semicircular canal occlusion: a safe and highly effective treatment for benign paroxysmal positional vertigo and superior canal dehiscence. Laryngoscope 2012;122(8):1862–6.
13. De Ridder D, Vanneste S, Engineer ND, et al. Safety and efficacy of vagus nerve stimulation paired with tones for the treatment of tinnitus: a case series. Neuromodulation 2014;17(2):170–9.
14. Lehtimäki J, Hyvärinen P, Ylikoski M, et al. Transcutaneous vagus nerve stimulation in tinnitus: a pilot study. Acta Otolaryngol 2013;133(4):378–82.
15. Kreuzer PM, Landgrebe M, Resch M, et al. Feasibility, safety and efficacy of transcutaneous vagus nerve stimulation in chronic tinnitus: an open pilot study. Brain Stimul 2014;7(5):740–7.
16. Lefaucheur JP, André-Obadia N, Antal A, et al. Evidence-based guidelines on the therapeutic use of repetitive transcranial magnetic stimulation (rTMS). Clin Neurophysiol 2014;125(11): 2150–206.
17. Cheung SW, Larson PS. Tinnitus modulation by deep brain stimulation in locus of caudate neurons (area LC). Neuroscience 2010;169(4):1768–78.
18. Shi Y, Burchiel KJ, Anderson VC, et al. Deep brain stimulation effects in patients with tinnitus. Otolaryngol Head Neck Surg 2009;141(2):285–7.

19. Smit JV, Janssen ML, Schulze H, et al. Deep brain stimulation in tinnitus: current and future perspectives. Brain Res 2015;1608:51–65.

20. Ramos Macías Á, Falcón González JC, Manrique M, et al. Cochlear implants as a treatment option for unilateral hearing loss, severe tinnitus and hyperacusis. Audiol Neurootol 2015;20(Suppl 1):60–6.

21. Punte AK, Vermeire K, Hofkens A, et al. Cochlear implantation as a durable tinnitus treatment in single-sided deafness. Cochlear Implants Int 2011; 12(Suppl 1):S26–9.

22. Tyler RS, Keiner AJ, Walker K, et al. A series of case studies of tinnitus suppression with mixed background stimuli in a cochlear implant. Am J Audiol 2015;24(3):398–410.

23. Lavigne P, Lavigne F, Saliba I. Intratympanic corticosteroids injections: a systematic review of literature. Eur Arch Otorhinolaryngol 2015;1–8 [Epub ahead of print].

24. Shim HJ, Song SJ, Choi AY, et al. Comparison of various treatment modalities for acute tinnitus. Laryngoscope 2011;121(12):2619–25.

25. Hidaka H, Honkura Y, Ota J, et al. Middle ear myoclonus cured by selective tenotomy of the tensor tympani: strategies for targeted intervention for middle ear muscles. Otol Neurotol 2013;34(9):1552–8.

26. Bhimrao SK, Masterson L, Baguley D. Systematic review of management strategies for middle ear myoclonus. Otolaryngol Head Neck Surg 2012. http://dx.doi.org/10.1177/0194599811434504.

27. Adil E, Poe D. What is the full range of medical and surgical treatments available for patients with eustachian tube dysfunction? Curr Opin Otolaryngol Head Neck Surg 2014;22(1):8–15.

28. Hussein AA, Adams AS, Turner JH. Surgical management of patulous eustachian tube: a systematic review. Laryngoscope 2015;125(9):2193–8.

29. Berguer R, Nowak P. Treatment of venous pulsatile tinnitus in younger women. Ann Vasc Surg 2015; 29(4):650–3.

30. Bae SC, Kim DK, Yeo SW, et al. Single-center 10-year experience in treating patients with vascular tinnitus: diagnostic approaches and treatment outcomes. Clin Exp Otorhinolaryngol 2015;8(1):7–12.

31. Jackler RK, Brackmann DE, Sismanis A. A warning on venous ligation for pulsatile tinnitus. Otol Neurotol 2001;22(3):427–8.

32. Harvey RS, Hertzano R, Kelman SE, et al. Pulse-synchronous tinnitus and sigmoid sinus wall anomalies: descriptive epidemiology and the idiopathic intracranial hypertension patient population. Otol Neurotol 2014;35(1):7–15.

33. Dong C, Zhao PF, Yang JG, et al. Incidence of vascular anomalies and variants associated with unilateral venous pulsatile tinnitus in 242 patients based on dual-phase contrast-enhanced computed tomography. Chin Med J 2015;128(5):581.

34. Grewal AK, Kim HY, Comstock RH, et al. Clinical presentation and imaging findings in patients with pulsatile tinnitus and sigmoid sinus diverticulum/dehiscence. Otol Neurotol 2014;35(1):16–21.

35. Schoeff S, Nicholas B, Mukherjee S, et al. Imaging prevalence of sigmoid sinus dehiscence among patients with and without pulsatile tinnitus. Otolaryngol Head Neck Surg 2014. http://dx.doi.org/10.1177/0194599813520291.

36. Comstock RH III, Grewal AK, Wycherly BJ. Surgical resolution of pulsatile tinnitus from sigmoid sinus diverticulum/dehiscence. 116th Annual Meeting of the Triological Society. Orlando, FL, USA, April 12–13, 2013.

37. Liu Z, Dong C, Wang X, et al. Association between idiopathic intracranial hypertension and sigmoid sinus dehiscence/diverticulum with pulsatile tinnitus: a retrospective imaging study. Neuroradiology 2015;57(7):747–53.

38. Houdart E, Chapot R, Merland JJ. Aneurysm of a dural sigmoid sinus: a novel vascular cause of pulsatile tinnitus. Ann Neurol 2000;48(4):669–71.

39. Sanchez TG, Murao M, de Medeiros IR, et al. A new therapeutic procedure for treatment of objective venous pulsatile tinnitus. Int Tinnitus J 2002;8(1): 54–7.

40. Zenteno M, Murillo-Bonilla L, Martínez S, et al. Endovascular treatment of a transverse-sigmoid sinus aneurysm presenting as pulsatile tinnitus: case report. J Neurosurg 2004;100(1):120–2.

41. Otto KJ, Hudgins PA, Abdelkafy W, et al. Sigmoid sinus diverticulum: a new surgical approach to the correction of pulsatile tinnitus. Otol Neurotol 2007; 28(1):48–53.

42. Eisenman DJ. Sinus wall reconstruction for sigmoid sinus diverticulum and dehiscence: a standardized surgical procedure for a range of radiographic findings. Otol Neurotol 2011;32(7):1116–9.

43. Geng W, Liu Z, Fan Z. CT characteristics of dehiscent sigmoid plates presenting as pulsatile tinnitus: a study of 23 patients. Acta Radiol 2014. http://dx.doi.org/10.1177/0284185114559762.

44. Guo P, Wang WQ. Degree of sigmoid sinus compression and the symptom relief using magnetic resonance angiography in venous pulsating tinnitus. Clin Exp Otorhinolaryngol 2015;8(2):111–6.

45. Raghavan P, Serulle Y. Postoperative imaging findings following sigmoid sinus wall reconstruction for pulse synchronous tinnitus. AJNR Am J Neuroradiol 2016 Jan;37(1):136–42.

Endovascular Interventions for Idiopathic Intracranial Hypertension and Venous Tinnitus: New Horizons

Ferdinand K. Hui, MD[a],*, Todd Abruzzo, MD[b],
Sameer A. Ansari, MD, PhD[c,d,e]

KEYWORDS

- Venous tinnitus • Intracranial hypertension • Endovascular intervention

KEY POINTS

- Pulsatile tinnitus from intracranial venous abnormalities is an uncommon and increasingly recognized cause of pulse synchronous tinnitus.
- Venous Stenoses associated with idiopathic intracranial hypertension can be treated with venous sinus stenting though randomized data is lacking.
- Venous abnormalities such as venous diverticulae or fenestrations may rarely cause venous tinnitus, and in select cases, may be successfully treated with venous embolization or stenting.

BACKGROUND

The term tinnitus describes a subjective ringing or buzzing in the ear, which may be continuous or pulsatile. Vascular causes of symptomatic, pulsatile tinnitus may include arterial variant anatomy (aberrant internal carotid artery, persistent stapedial artery, neurovascular loop compression syndromes); high-flow arterial diseases, including hypervascular tumors (glomus jugulare or tympanicum); arteriovenous shunt lesions (dural arteriovenous fistula or arteriovenous malformations of the head and neck); and arterial diseases of the head and neck associated with turbulence or flow acceleration (pseudoaneurysms and stenoses related to dissection, atherosclerotic vascular disease, or fibromuscular dysplasia). Venous causes of tinnitus

are less well described and may result from congenital or acquired venous anomalies of the jugular bulb or sigmoid sinus (dehiscence, diverticula, aneurysms, fenestrations, webs) or stenoses of the dural venous sinuses (transverse and/ or sigmoid sinus), including those associated with idiopathic intracranial hypertension (IIH).[1]

The management of tinnitus remains complex, and a recent review of available randomized data regarding medical management of nonpulsatile tinnitus suggest that data is insufficient for best practice guidelines.[2] An older review by Dobie and colleagues[3] is similar in that the primary focus was nonpulsatile tinnitus, and that venous tinnitus was not described in terms of treatment protocols. Venous causes of tinnitus may also be sufficiently

Disclosures: None.
[a] Department of Radiology, Johns Hopkins University, Baltimore, MD 21287, USA; [b] Department of Neurosurgery, Mayfield Clinic and Cincinnati Children's Hospital, University of Cincinnati, Cincinnati, OH 45209, USA; [c] Department of Radiology, Northwestern University, IL 60611, USA; [d] Department of Neurology, Northwestern University, IL 60611, USA; [e] Department of Neurological Surgery, Northwestern University, IL 60611, USA
* Corresponding author.
E-mail address: fhui2@jhmi.edu

rare such that large-scale, randomized data may be difficult to obtain. Other than venous disease in the setting of intracranial hypertension, review of the literature regarding venous tinnitus shows it is marked with multiple small series and case reports.

VENOUS TINNITUS

Venous tinnitus is typically characterized as pulse synchronous and represents a smaller subset of tinnitus in general.[1] Unlike arterial causes of pulse synchronous tinnitus, tinnitus that is caused by venous disease or anomalous venous anatomy can be reduced or extinguished by direct jugular venous compression or by turning the head to the side. Pulsatile tinnitus caused by venous disease is aggravated by straining, bending, or Valsalva maneuvers. In contrast to patients with arterial-type pulsatile tinnitus, patients with venous-type pulsatile tinnitus learn that they can reduce or eliminate their tinnitus by sleeping with the affected side in a dependent position. Dural arteriovenous fistulas, lesions typically located in the dural venous sinuses, are high-flow arteriovenous shunt lesions that may also result in pulsatile tinnitus[4] of the arterial type. For detailed discussion of these lesions, (See Miller TR, Serulle Y, Gandhi D: Arterial abnormalities leading to tinnitus, in this issue.)

IDIOPATHIC INTRACRANIAL HYPERTENSION

Benign or idiopathic, intracranial hypertension (also known as pseudotumor cerebri) may present with adjunctive symptoms of venous tinnitus. In 1998, Sismanis,[5] published a 15-year experience of pulsatile tinnitus and noted 56 out of 145 subjects with tinnitus had a diagnosis of IIH. Forty of these subjects were classified as having objective tinnitus versus 16 with subjective tinnitus. In this series, as in other contemporaneous series, no proposed mechanism for tinnitus was mentioned. However, direct pressure on the ipsilateral jugular vein typically results in cessation of the pulsatile tinnitus, suggesting that this is a venous flow–related phenomenon.

Mechanism of Venous Stenosis and Venous Hypertension

The exact pathophysiology for IIH is unknown. It may be related to reduced cerebrospinal fluid (CSF) absorption or overproduction of CSF. It is thought that decreased CSF absorption may occur in the setting of venous hypertension and, as such, venous hypertension has been put forth as the inciting cause for IIH, with early animal experiments outlining the relationship of increased intracranial pressure and venous pressures.[6] Later work by Karahalios and colleagues[7] proposed that venous hypertension is a universal mechanism for IIH. They found elevated venous pressures in all subjects clinically diagnosed with IIH in their series. Increased venous pressures, intracranially and systemically, may be secondary to focal stenosis or venous outflow obstructions, as well as systemic venous hypertension, often associated with morbid obesity.[8] This may, in part, explain the preponderance of IIH in obese young women.

The presence of venous stenosis in these patients has been gradually recognized, with early work estimating venous outflow obstruction in 19.7% of cases in a series of 188 subjects followed clinically by Johnston and colleagues[9] for 3 decades. This study was hampered by lack of high-resolution assessment of the cervical and intracranial draining veins; a point conceded by the investigators. In 2003, Farb and colleagues[10] prospectively evaluated 29 subjects with clinically diagnosed IIH compared with 50 normal controls and found that significant bilateral venous stenoses were found in 27 out of 29 (93%) of the IIH subjects compared with 4 out of 59 (6%) in controls. Similarly, Rohr and colleagues[11] reported the presence of venous stenosis in the setting of IIH in a smaller series. It is likely that IIH-related venous tinnitus results from turbulent blood flow and flow acceleration across the regions of venous stenosis. However, the cause of venous stenosis remains obscure, though both venous thrombosis (endoluminal obstruction) and extrinsic compression (compression from elevated CSF pressures) have both been postulated. Indeed, there are reports of other processes, such as dural sinus thrombosis or partial thrombosis, as well as dural arteriovenous fistulas, resulting in venous outflow obstruction that have been associated with increased intracranial pressures and attendant symptoms.[12,13]

Clinical Management

The primary goal in managing patients with IIH is to avoid irreversible vision loss and reduce the intensity of headaches. A complete neurologic history and physical examination should be performed including a neuro-ophthalmology evaluation for objective assessment of vision, papilledema, and elevated intraocular pressures. IIH-associated optic neuropathy is a result of prolonged increased CSF pressure within the optic nerve sheath. Given the prevalence of morbid obesity in these patients, weight loss is considered as a first-line management option. Lifestyle modifications with caloric restriction,[14] as well as surgical weight loss strategies,[15] have been described in small series with reported effectiveness in controlling the symptoms of IIH. If weight loss cannot be achieved, medical management with carbonic anhydrase inhibitors should be considered. Acetazolamide[16] and topiramate[17] may be used to medically manage symptoms. Acetazolamide can reduce CSF production but also functions as a cerebral vasodilator to increase cerebral blood volume capacitance and potentially reduce the venous and CSF pressure gradients. However, carbonic anhydrase inhibitors may not be tolerated due to side effects (paresthesias, malaise, headaches) or contraindications (hypersensitivity to sulfonamides, electrolyte disturbances, renal or liver disease, adrenocortical insufficiency, and long-term use in chronic angle closure glaucoma).

To reduce the pernicious effect of chronic CSF hypertension, CSF diversion with ventriculoperitoneal shunts has been described and can effectively reduce symptoms of papilledema and headaches.[18] Optic nerve sheath fenestration results in perforation of the cranial nerve II nerve sheath, allowing CSF to flow out into the orbit, thereby locally reducing optic nerve pressures. This has been performed acutely as well as for more chronic presentations.[19,20] Clinical indications for intervention have focused on preserving vision rather than treatment of tinnitus and efficacy in terms of venous tinnitus treatment is unclear.

Endovascular Treatment Considerations

Accumulating experience suggests that endovascular treatment of venous stenoses associated with IIH may be an effective alternative to CSF diversion and optic nerve sheath fenestration. Moreover, tinnitus seems to resolve at a high rate in these reports. Intracranial stent placement across venous stenoses has been performed with good technical success rates[21–24] (**Fig. 1**). Ahmed and colleagues[25] described their experience with

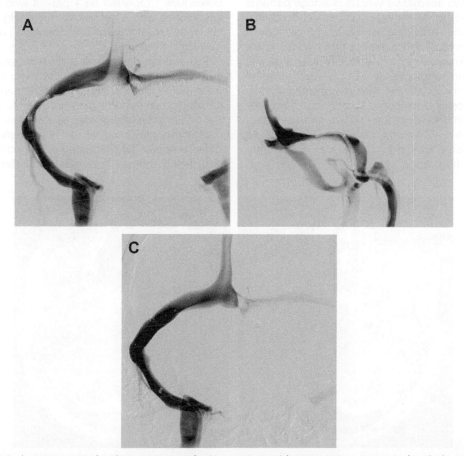

Fig. 1. Typical appearance of catheter venography in a patient with venous sinus stenosis. (*A, B*) The anteroposterior and lateral appearance of such a tapered narrowing. (*C*) After stent appearance with resolution of the venous stenosis and pressure gradient on manometry.

52 IIH subjects treated with endovascular stenting and reported resolution of mean pressure gradients of 20 mm Hg, improvement of symptoms attributable to intracranial hypertension and papilledema, and relapses in 6 subjects who were subsequently treated with stent revision. Tinnitus was reported in 17 out of 52 (32%) subjects with resolution in 100% after stenting. In a meta-analysis of endovascularly treated cases of IIH performed by Puffer and colleagues,[26] they reported the pooled results of 143 venous stenting subjects with 48% presenting with pulsatile tinnitus and high improvement rates (93%) after stent placement. Endovascular treatment of venous stenoses and associated tinnitus seems to be both safe and effective.

With respect to the technical procedure, treatment planning may be achieved by either noninvasive imaging through either gadolinium-enhanced MR venography (MRV) or computed tomography venography (CTV), or invasively using transarterial access to analyze the cerebral circulation, specifically the bilateral dural venous sinuses and alternative venous drainage patterns in the setting of venous stenosis and outflow obstruction, providing a treatment plan with road mapping capabilities for transvenous intervention. Three-dimensional (3D) rotational digital subtraction angiography (DSA) with delayed acquisitions to assess the venous phase may be an excellent adjunct to identify optimum projections that confirm the venous stenoses suspected on noninvasive imaging, as well as intervention planning for vessel sizing and stent selection (Fig. 2).

Procedures can be performed with the patient awake, under conscious sedation, or with general anesthesia, although general anesthesia may result in reduction of observed gradients and stenoses (Ferdinand Hui, Mark Luciano, personal communication, 2014). Indeed, any of these pharmacologic agents may have an effect on venous pressure measurements. Transvenous access requires either femoral or direct internal jugular venous access for stable sheath support, especially if venous sinus stenting will be performed in the same setting. Aggressive intraprocedural anticoagulation with heparin is recommended (Activated Clotting Time 2–2.5x baseline or 250–300 seconds) to avoid venous thrombosis complications in this low-flow vasculature. Before intervention, most investigators report the use of manometry proximal and distal to the venous stenosis to establish the presence of a pressure gradient but with continued uncertainty as to the proper treatment threshold.[23,24] In the review by Arac and colleagues,[23] the gradients measured ranged between 8 and 43 mm Hg. Radvany and colleagues[22] reported on 1 patient who received intervention with a gradient of 5 mm Hg but with intravascular ultrasound documentation of intraluminal filling defects.

The authors have used a pressure gradient of 8 mm Hg as an adequate indication for endovascular therapy to prevent secondary complications of intracranial hypertension. In patients in whom the primary clinical concern is intolerable tinnitus, manometry may be of secondary importance. All patients should be pretreated or loaded with dual antiplatelet therapy if venous sinus stenting will

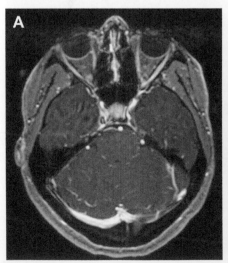
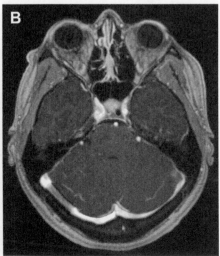

Fig. 2. (A) Postcontrast spoiled gradient MR angiography with a narrowed segment of linear enhancement sinus corresponding to the venous stenosis in the right transverse. (B) Typical appearance after stent placement with subtle regions of susceptibility artifact along the column of contrast and resolution of the focal stenosis.

be performed. Typically, carotid-type self-expanding stents are used for venous sinus stenting as an off-label application. Appropriate stent sizing should account for the native size of the highly compliant dural venous sinus with 10% to 20% oversizing for stable deployment and apposition to the vessel wall; however, grossly oversized stents may result in temporary worsening of headaches, possibly related to dural irritation (Hui, personal communication, 2014; Gailloud, personal communication, 2013). The stiffness of carotid stents may be result in difficulty advancing the stent through the tortuous intracranial dural venous sinuses and may require additional support with flexible guide sheaths and extensive microguidewire (0.014–0.018 in) support into the contralateral transverse-sigmoid or sagittal sinuses, or even the contralateral internal jugular vein. Larger guidewires are sometimes necessary for adequate support but should be deployed with caution due to the risk of dural venous sinus perforation and errant passage into cerebral veins, which are relatively fragile and prone to perforation. Care is required in superselective catheterization and advancement of the rigid stent delivery catheters to prevent injury to the ostia of the draining tributary veins, such as the vein of Labbé. Postprocedure angiography and manometry should confirm the resolution of the venous stenosis and the associated pressure gradient across the stent construct with no evidence of poor stent apposition, stent migration, significant residual stenosis, or in-stent thrombosis.

OTHER CAUSES OF VENOUS TINNITUS AMENABLE TO ENDOVASCULAR INTERVENTIONS

Waldvogel and colleagues[27] performed a review of 84 subjects with pulsatile tinnitus using noninvasive ultrasound, CT angiography, and MR imaging, as well as conventional angiography, to diagnose the sources of tinnitus. They reported that 36 subjects (42%) harbored arterial disease (dissections, aneurysms, arteriovenous fistulas); 12%, nonvascular disease (glomus tumors and intracranial hypertension); 14%, venous disease (venous anomalies and thrombosis or stenosis); and 27 (32%), unknown causes. In addition, Sonmez and colleagues[28] studied a series of 74 subjects presenting with pulsatile tinnitus and detected relevant disease with noninvasive imaging in 50 (67.6%). They reported the most common cause as a high jugular bulb (21%) followed by atherosclerosis, dehiscent jugular bulbs, aneurysms of internal carotid artery, dural arteriovenous

fistula, aberrant internal carotid artery, jugular diverticulum, and glomus tumor.

Venous sources of tinnitus include

1. Venous anomalies
2. Venous aneurysms or diverticula (jugular or sigmoid sinus dehiscence)
3. Venous stenosis or intracranial hypertension.

In general, venous tinnitus arises from vibrations (initiated by turbulent or accelerated intravascular flow) conducted to the adjacent labyrinth and cochlea, resulting in a pulse-synchronous character.[1] Historically, venous tinnitus has been treated with ipsilateral jugular vein ligation[1,29,30] but more recently with endovascular therapies.[31,32]

IMAGING OF VENOUS TINNITUS

Before the presumptive treatment of venous sources of tinnitus, careful cross-sectional imaging evaluation, especially of the temporal bones and skull base, should be performed via high-resolution bone algorithm CT and/or MR imaging to exclude hypervascular tumors and other causes, such as hemosiderosis affecting cranial nerves.[33,34] CT or MR angiography is usually sufficient to identify anatomic arterial variants or other diseases, though screening for dural arteriovenous fistula has traditionally been approached with catheter angiography. Recently, improving time-resolved MR imaging and dynamic CT angiography techniques have allowed the diagnosis of arteriovenous shunt lesions. Nonetheless, the sensitivity and specificity of the novel approaches have not been adequately characterized and their limitations are incompletely understood. Consequently, the authors still rely on DSA to exclude dural arteriovenous shunt disease.[35,36] If venous tinnitus is still suspected, CTV or MRV techniques can be very useful for diagnostic screening or even endovascular or surgical treatment planning as an adjunct to catheter angiography or venography.

Using cross-sectional techniques, such as CTV-MRV, multiplanar capabilities, gadolinium, or iodine-based contrast blood pool effect, enhances venous opacification compared with DSA. DSA–DS venography with 3D delayed acquisition, however, uses longer bolus and delay in acquisition and, therefore, can maximize opacification of venous structures. These acquisitions may also provide cross-sectional data.

ABERRANT VENOUS ANATOMY

Given the structural nature of venous tinnitus, aberrant condylar or mastoid emissary veins that course near the cochlear apparatus may be responsible for venous tinnitus. Lambert and Cantrell[37] described an aberrant posterior condylar emissary vein that was associated with pulsatile tinnitus. Venous sinus fenestrations are anecdotally reported to be associated with tinnitus (**Fig. 3**).

Endovascular Treatment Considerations

Endovascular treatment of congenital venous abnormalities has not been well described and no significant data exist. Although the aim of treatment may be to disconnect aberrant veins with occlusive agents, eliminating conducted pulsatile vibrations to the inner ear, the resulting alterations in normal venous drainage could result in venous thrombosis and venous hypertension complications such as ischemia, hemorrhage, and intracranial hypertension. Embolic agents should be sized to the vessel of interest and detachable coils are primarily chosen to eliminate abnormal emissary veins. Detachable coils are preferred to liquid embolic agents due to their controllable detachment to prevent venous migration. Experience with fenestrations and webs is limited and stent reconstruction may be considered, with the cautionary note that inadvertent reduction of venous outflow may result in venous hypertension. Analogous to venous diverticula or dehiscence lesions, preoperative testing across these venous variants should be performed before intervention with balloon occlusion or venous pressure measurements to ascertain a functional or hemodynamic impairment related to the venous anomaly.

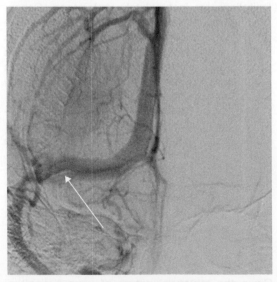

Fig. 3. Catheter venography in a patient with pulsatile tinnitus ipsilateral to a transverse sinus fenestration, ostensibly the source of tinnitus.

HIGH-RIDING JUGULAR FOSSA

The high-riding jugular bulb or fossa describes cases in which the jugular fossa is anatomically situated higher in the skull base, abutting the sigmoid plate adjacent to the mastoid air cells and, occasionally, in direct contact with the cochlea. A high-riding jugular bulb may or may not be associated with diverticula (Stern 1980) and/or osseous dehiscence. This abnormality is thought to be related to tinnitus due to abnormal conduction into the temporal bone and cochlea. Wadin and colleagues[38] evaluated 112 temporal bones with high jugular fossa and identified 43 jugular bulb diverticula. However, only 2 subjects had tinnitus and vertigo and 3 subjects had hearing loss. In this series, when the cochlea was located in close proximity to the jugular fossa (3 subjects), all presented with tinnitus.

Couloigner and colleagues[39] describe a series of 13 subjects with concomitant Meniere disease, high-riding jugular bulb, vertigo, and pulsatile tinnitus. The subjects were treated with complete mastoidectomy and repositioning of the jugular bulb via an infralabyrinthine and subfacial approach, displacing the bulb with surgical wax. In the subjects treated with surgery, disabling vertigo diminished from 12 (92%) to 1 (8%) with reduction in tinnitus in 4 (31%) and resolution in 3 (23%).

Surgical ligation of the ipsilateral jugular vein has been described as an effective treatment of these lesions.[29,30] Endovascular techniques were reported by Signorelli and colleagues.[32]

Endovascular Treatment Considerations

Endovascular treatment should be considered in conjunction with otolaryngology consultation, balancing the potential risks and benefits of treatment by endovascular occlusion against those associated with mastoid reconstruction and jugular repositioning, which is arguably more invasive. The objective of endovascular therapy is to eliminate flow through the high jugular fossa by embolic occlusion. Complete jugular occlusion, even extracranially, may be able to achieve cessation of tinnitus in a similar manner to open surgical ligation but segmental occlusion of the fossa itself may be preferable. Endovascular occlusion of the jugular vein can be accomplished with several endovascular devices such as detachable balloons; a nest of metal fibers, such as the Amplatzer vascular occlusion device (St Jude, St, Paul, MN, USA); or oversized detachable coils with or without adjunctive stenting of the venous sinus to stabilize the endovenous coil mass.

Both endovascular and surgical ligation of the offending jugular vein may result in venous outflow obstruction. Cervical and/or intracranial venous hypertension may result if there are insufficient venous collateral routes or the contralateral sinus anatomy and jugular venous drainage is hypoplastic and inadequate. Careful evaluation of cerebral venous outflow is mandatory before jugular vein sacrifice. Signorelli and colleagues[32] raise the concern of venous hypertension in patients with insufficient intracranial venous drainage after jugular sacrifice and the possibility of pulmonary emboli from the occluded venous stump. Additionally, Jackler and colleagues[40] reported thromboemboli status after internal jugular vein occlusion.

VENOUS DIVERTICULA, DEHISCENCE, AND/ OR ANEURYSMS

The language describing venous diverticula in the literature is ambiguous and inconsistent. The authors regard this category to be inclusive of any focal outpouching of the major intratemporal venous structures, such as the sigmoid sinus or jugular bulb. Dehiscence refers to a segment of absent bone with diverticulum or without herniation of vein or venous material through the osseous defect (Figs. 4 and 5). These lesions are also thought to result in tinnitus due to turbulent flow within the pouch. Grewal and colleagues[41] analyzed CT temporal bone findings in 61 subjects with pulsatile tinnitus compared with a consecutive cohort of 200 controls. In the control group, 35 subjects (18%) possessed incidental sigmoid sinus diverticulum-dehiscence. On subsequent history taking, 12 out of 35 of the control subjects with dehiscence (34%) complained of pulsatile tinnitus. Conversely, in 61 subjects with pulsatile tinnitus, 15 (25%) harbored sigmoid sinus diverticulum-dehiscence. The investigators go on to state that sigmoid sinus diverticula and dehiscence may be the most common cause of venous tinnitus given the prevalence in both their controls and study group.

Successful surgical reconstruction of these lesions has been reported by multiple investigators. Otto and colleagues[42] noted similar results in their series. In 3 of 5 subjects with sigmoid sinus diverticula and no other discernible causes of tinnitus, transmastoid surgical reconstruction eliminated the tinnitus. Thirteen subjects treated in a series by Eisenman[43] underwent 14 transmastoid reconstructions of both sigmoid sinus diverticula and dehiscence, reporting excellent resolution of their tinnitus.

Open neurosurgical treatment has also been described that uses open surgical craniectomy and coagulation[44] to cure a transverse-sigmoid sinus venous aneurysm-diverticulum presenting with pulsatile tinnitus. Jugular diverticula have been reported to be a risk factor for iatrogenic hemorrhage during middle ear surgery. Shihada and colleagues[45] reported a pediatric patient who experienced severe hemorrhage after myringotomy and was successfully treated with endovascular occlusion of the lesion.

Endovascular Treatment Considerations

Endovascular treatment of diverticula, aneurysms, or dehiscence allows occlusion of the lesion, buffering the inflow vibrations conducted to the cochlea. Houdart and colleagues[46] describe an outpouching of the sigmoid sinus that was treated with endovascular occlusion of the diverticulum using detachable coils. Gard and colleagues[47] also reported successful coil embolization in a single patient with a symptomatic venous diverticulum resulting in resolution of tinnitus. Meanwhile, Park and colleagues[48] described awake embolization of a sigmoid sinus diverticulum in a 31-year-old woman with a right temporal bone dehiscence. During coil embolization with 2 detachable coils, the patient reported cessation of tinnitus, leading to the completion of the procedure. The awake approach allowed immediate confirmation of treatment efficacy.

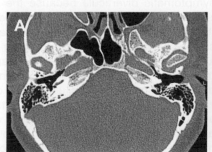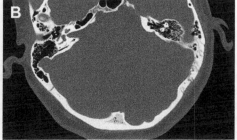

Fig. 4. (A, B) Typical CT imaging of 2 patients with sigmoid plate thinning or dehiscence without diverticula. The patients both presented with pulsatile tinnitus.

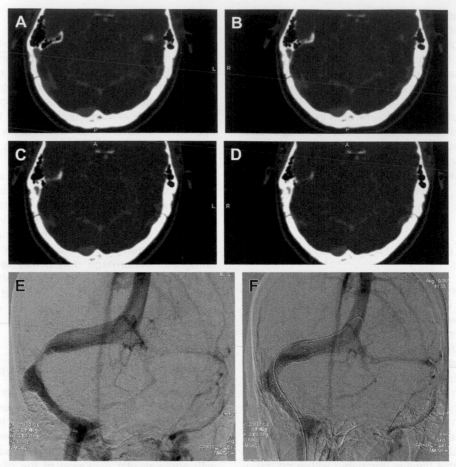

Fig. 5. (*A–D*) CT imaging of a patient with a sigmoid sinus diverticulum in serial axial images. (*E, F*) Catheter venography before and after stent placement across a venous stenosis in a patient with both IIH and a sigmoid diverticulum, with patient experiencing resolution of symptoms after stenting.

Zenteno and colleagues[49] treated a transverse-sigmoid sinus aneurysm with stenting; however, the stent alone did not result in tinnitus cessation and follow-up coiling was performed for cure. Sigmoid sinus diverticula-dehiscence is often associated with upstream venous stenoses. It has been proposed that the flow jet engendered by the stenosis impinges on the wall of the sigmoid sinus, resulting in shear-related mural weakening of the venous sinus and dehiscence of underlying bone. The association has been seen in cases of IIH (Fig. 4). Reports have suggested treatment of the stenosis and the diverticulum may be required for efficacy.

However, a recent case report by Amans and colleagues[50] specifically targeted a large sigmoid sinus diverticulum with coil embolization without stenting the associated upstream venous stenosis, resulting in resolution of pulsatile tinnitus.

Endovascular approaches for these lesions are not without risk. Sanchez and colleagues[51] reported a small area of cerebellar ischemia after embolization of a sigmoid sinus diverticulum with the ataxia resolving over 2 months back to baseline. The ischemic complication was likely related to endovascular occlusion of a cerebellar tributary vein associated with the diverticulum during embolization.

Transvenous coil embolization of a diverticulum may be the primary treatment option for symptomatic diverticula because the approach is less invasive than open surgical options. If the neck of the lesion does not adequately allow stable coil placement, stents may be used adjunctively but do require extended antiplatelet therapy for 3 to 6 months to prevent in-stent thrombosis complications until stent endothelization can occur. Given the size of the sigmoid sinus, standard intracranial stents diameters are inadequate, and biliary or carotid stents must be considered. Although it is conceivable that some diverticula or dehiscence may become asymptomatic by stent therapy alone, there is currently no experience to support this approach.

In the case of dehiscence without herniation, in which there is no diverticulum sac for embolization, sacrifice of the venous structure can be considered. As previously discussed, when treating high-riding jugular bulbs, the patient's cerebral venous outflow capacity and the invasiveness of surgical reconstruction should be carefully balanced. Surgical options involving reconstruction of the sigmoid plate may be considered as superior alternatives to deconstructive endovascular approaches in this particular setting.

SUMMARY

Pulsatile tinnitus from intracranial venous abnormalities is an uncommon but increasingly recognized cause of pulse synchronous tinnitus. These symptoms are related to flow turbulence in normal or anomalous venous structures, be they high-riding jugular bulbs, anatomic variants, osseous dehiscence, diverticula, aneurysms, or venous stenoses conducted to the adjacent cochlea. Many of these lesions can be approached using surgical or endovascular techniques that aim to eliminate flow through the abnormal structure (in the case of ligation or embolization), or repositioning of the offending structure. Endovascular therapies may have applications in many of these disease conditions. They have the advantage of being minimally invasive and may selectively eliminate the site of turbulence.

Most experience in the treatment of venous stenoses for tinnitus has been performed for lesions associated with IIH. Stenting has been used successfully to treat venous stenoses with low complication rates and high success rates. At present, randomized controlled data are lacking. Careful exclusion of other causes of tinnitus should be performed before consideration for surgical or endovascular treatment of presumed causative lesions.

REFERENCES

1. Chandler JR. Diagnosis and cure of venous hum tinnitus. Laryngoscope 1983;93(7):892–5.
2. Hoare DJ, Kowalkowski VL, Kang S, et al. Systematic review and meta-analyses of randomized controlled trials examining tinnitus management. Laryngoscope 2011;121(7):1555–64.
3. Dobie RA. A review of randomized clinical trials in tinnitus. Laryngoscope 1999;109(8):1202–11.
4. Shah SB, Lalwani AK, Dowd CF. Transverse/sigmoid sinus dural arteriovenous fistulas presenting as pulsatile tinnitus. Laryngoscope 1999;109(1):54–8.

5. Sismanis A. Pulsatile tinnitus. A 15-year experience. Am J Otol 1998;19(4):472–7.
6. Johnston IH, Rowan JO. Raised intracranial pressure and cerebral blood flow 3. Venous outflow tract pressures and vascular resistances in experimental intracranial hypertension. J Neurol Neurosurg Psychiatry 1974;37(4):392–402.
7. Karahalios DG, Rekate HL, Khayata MH, et al. Elevated intracranial venous pressure as a universal mechanism in pseudotumor cerebri of varying etiologies. Neurology 1996;46(1):198–202.
8. Sugerman HJ, DeMaria EJ, Felton W, et al. Increased intra-abdominal pressure and cardiac filling pressures in obesity-associated pseudotumor cerebri. Neurology 1997;49(2):507–11.
9. Johnston I, Kollar C, Dunkley S, et al. Cranial venous outflow obstruction in the pseudotumour syndrome: incidence, nature and relevance. J Clin Neurosci 2002;9(3):273–8.
10. Farb RI, Vanek I, Scott JN, et al. Idiopathic intracranial hypertension the prevalence and morphology of sinovenous stenosis. Neurology 2003;60(9):1418–24.
11. Rohr A, Dörner L, Stingele R, et al. Reversibility of venous sinus obstruction in idiopathic intracranial hypertension. AJNR Am J Neuroradiol 2007;28(4):656–9.
12. Biousse V, Ameri A, Bousser MG. Isolated intracranial hypertension as the only sign of cerebral venous thrombosis. Neurology 1999;53(7):1537–42.
13. Cognard C, Casasco A, Toevi M, et al. Dural arteriovenous fistulas as a cause of intracranial hypertension due to impairment of cranial venous outflow. J Neurol Neurosurg Psychiatry 1998;65(3):308–16.
14. Sinclair AJ, Burdon MA, Nightingale PG, et al. Low energy diet and intracranial pressure in women with idiopathic intracranial hypertension: prospective cohort study. BMJ 2010;341:c270.
15. Sugerman HJ, Felton WL III, Sismanis A, et al. Gastric surgery for pseudotumor cerebri associated with severe obesity. Ann Surg 1999;229(5):634.
16. Johnson LN, Krohel GB, Madsen RW, et al. The role of weight loss and acetazolamide in the treatment of idiopathic intracranial hypertension (pseudotumor cerebri). Ophthalmology 1998;105(12):2313–7.
17. Alore PL, Jay WM, Macken MP. Topiramate, pseudotumor cerebri, weight-loss and glaucoma: an ophthalmologic perspective. In: Seminars in ophthalmology, vol. 21. United Kingdom: Informa UK Ltd; 2006. p. 15–7. No. 1.
18. Rosenberg ML, Corbett JJ, Smith C, et al. Cerebrospinal fluid diversion procedures in pseudotumor cerebri. Neurology 1993;43(6):1071–2.
19. Thambisetty M, Lavin PJ, Newman NJ, et al. Fulminant idiopathic intracranial hypertension. Neurology 2007;68(3):229–32.
20. Agarwal MR, Yoo JH. Optic nerve sheath fenestration for vision preservation in idiopathic intracranial hypertension. Neurosurg Focus 2007;23(5):E7.

21. Owler BK, Parker G, Halmagyi GM, et al. Pseudotumor cerebri syndrome: venous sinus obstruction and its treatment with stent placement. J Neurosurg 2003;98(5):1045–55.

22. Radvany MG, Solomon D, Nijjar S, et al. Visual and neurological outcomes following endovascular stenting for pseudotumor cerebri associated with transverse sinus stenosis. J Neuroophthalmol 2013;33(2):117–22.

23. Arac A, Lee M, Steinberg GK, et al. Efficacy of endovascular stenting in dural venous sinus stenosis for the treatment of idiopathic intracranial hypertension. Neurosurg Focus 2009;27(5):E14.

24. Owler BK, Parker G, Halmagyi GM, et al. Cranial venous outflow obstruction and pseudotumor cerebri syndrome. In: Pickard JD, editor. Advances and technical standards in neurosurgery. Vienna (Austria): Springer; 2005. p. 107–74.

25. Ahmed RM, Wilkinson M, Parker GD, et al. Transverse sinus stenting for idiopathic intracranial hypertension: a review of 52 patients and of model predictions. AJNR Am J Neuroradiol 2011;32(8):1408–14.

26. Puffer RC, Mustafa W, Lanzino G. Venous sinus stenting for idiopathic intracranial hypertension: a review of the literature. J Neurointerv Surg 2013;5(5):483–6.

27. Waldvogel D, Mattle HP, Sturzenegger M, et al. Pulsatile tinnitus—a review of 84 patients. J Neurol 1998;245(3):137–42.

28. Sonmez G, Basekim CC, Ozturk E, et al. Imaging of pulsatile tinnitus: a review of 74 patients. Clin Imaging 2007;31(2):102–8.

29. Ward PH, Babin R, Calcaterra TC, et al. Operative treatment of surgical lesions with objective tinnitus. Ann Otol Rhinol Laryngol 1975;84(4):473–82.

30. Golueke PJ, Panetta T, Sclafani S, et al. Tinnitus originating from an abnormal jugular bulb: treatment by jugular vein ligation. J Vasc Surg 1987;6(3):248–51.

31. Mehanna R, Shaltoni H, Morsi H, et al. Endovascular treatment of sigmoid sinus aneurysm presenting as devastating pulsatile tinnitus a case report and review of literature. Interv Neuroradiol 2010;16(4):451–4.

32. Signorelli F, Mahla K, Turjman F. Endovascular treatment of two concomitant causes of pulsatile tinnitus: sigmoid sinus stenosis and ipsilateral jugular bulb diverticulum. Case report and literature review. Acta Neurochir (Wien) 2012;154(1):89–92.

33. Weekamp HH, Huygen PL, Merx JL, et al. Longitudinal analysis of hearing loss in a case of hemosiderosis of the central nervous system. Otol Neurotol 2003;24(5):738–42.

34. Weissman JL, Hirsch BE. Imaging of tinnitus: a review. Radiology 2000;216(2):342–9.

35. Narvid J, Do HM, Blevins NH, et al. CT angiography as a screening tool for dural arteriovenous fistula in patients with pulsatile tinnitus: feasibility and test characteristics. AJNR Am J Neuroradiol 2011;32:446–53.

36. Meckel S, Maier M, Ruiz DS, et al. MR angiography of dural arteriovenous fistulas: diagnosis and follow-up after treatment using a time-resolved 3D contrast-enhanced technique. AJNR Am J Neuroradiol 2007;28(5):877–84.

37. Lambert PR, Cantrell RW. Objective tinnitus in association with an abnormal posterior condylar emissary vein. Am J Otol 1986;7:204–7.

38. Wadin K, Thomander L, Wilbrand H. Effects of a high jugular fossa and jugular bulb diverticulum on the inner ear a clinical and radiologic investigation. Acta Radiol Diagn (Stockh) 1986;27(6):629–36.

39. Couloigner V, Grayeli AB, Bouccara D, et al. Surgical treatment of the high jugular bulb in patients with Meniere's disease and pulsatile tinnitus. Eur Arch Otorhinolaryngol 1999;256(5):224–9.

40. Jackler RK, Brackmann DE, Sismanis A. A warning on venous ligation for pulsatile tinnitus. Otol Neurotol 2001;22:427–8.

41. Grewal AK, Kim HY, Comstock RH III, et al. Clinical presentation and imaging findings in patients with pulsatile tinnitus and sigmoid sinus diverticulum/dehiscence. Otol Neurotol 2014;35(1):16–21.

42. Otto KJ, Hudgins PA, Abdelkafy W, et al. Sigmoid sinus diverticulum: a new surgical approach to the correction of pulsatile tinnitus. Otol Neurotol 2007;28(1):48–53.

43. Eisenman DJ. Sinus wall reconstruction for sigmoid sinus diverticulum and dehiscence: a standardized surgical procedure for a range of radiographic findings. Otol Neurotol 2011;32(7):1116–9.

44. Gologorsky Y, Meyer SA, Post AF, et al. Novel surgical treatment of a transverse-sigmoid sinus aneurysm presenting as pulsatile tinnitus: technical case report. Neurosurgery 2009;64(2):E393–4.

45. Shihada R, Maimon S, Braun J, et al. Endovascular embolization of a hemorrhagic jugular bulb diverticulum. Int J Pediatr Otorhinolaryngol 2008;72(9):1445–8.

46. Houdart E, Chapot R, Merland JJ. Aneurysm of a dural sigmoid sinus: a novel vascular cause of pulsatile tinnitus. Ann Neurol 2000;48:669–71.

47. Gard AP, Klopper HB, Thorell WE. Successful endovascular treatment of pulsatile tinnitus caused by a sigmoid sinus aneurysm a case report and review of the literature. Interv Neuroradiol 2009;15(4):425–8.

48. Park YH, Kwon HJ. Awake embolization of sigmoid sinus diverticulum causing pulsatile tinnitus: simultaneous confirmative diagnosis and treatment. Interv Neuroradiol 2011;17(3):376–9.

49. Zenteno M, Murillo-Bonilla L, Martínez S, et al. Endo-vascular treatment of a transverse-sigmoid sinus aneurysm presenting as pulsatile tinnitus: case report. J Neurosurg 2004;100(1):120–2.

50. Amans MR, Stout C, Dowd CF, et al. Resolution of pulsatile tinnitus after coil embolization of sigmoid sinus diverticulum. Austin J Cerebrovasc Dis Stroke 2014;1(2):1–3.

51. Sanchez TG, Murao M, de Medeiros IR, et al. A new therapeutic procedure for treatment of objective venous pulsatile tinnitus. Int Tinnitus J 2002;8(1): 54–7.

Advanced Neuroimaging of Tinnitus

Prashant Raghavan, MBBS[a,*], Andrew Steven, MD[a], Tanya Rath, MD[b],
Dheeraj Gandhi, MBBS, MD[c,d]

KEYWORDS

- Tinnitus • Neural networks • Functional MR imaging • Diffusion tensor imaging • Meniere disease
- Dural arteriovenous fistulae

KEY POINTS

- Tinnitus is associated with complex alterations to primary auditory, sensory, and limbic networks.
- Functional MR imaging and diffusion tensor imaging are capable of revealing such changes. This may aid in the identification of neural targets amenable to modification by novel treatment strategies.
- Newer MR imaging techniques that depict changes to the labyrinth in Meniere disease have emerged and may be of value in diagnosis in equivocal cases.
- Advances in computed tomography and MR imaging techniques have improved the ability to non-invasively diagnose dural arteriovenous fistulae.

INTRODUCTION

Previous articles have mostly dealt with the use of imaging techniques in the evaluation of structural causes of tinnitus. However, in most tinnitus sufferers, whose symptoms are subjective, routine imaging studies are unrevealing. It is now well known that complex alterations in auditory and nonauditory neural circuits underlie the genesis and perception of tinnitus and its associated symptoms in such patients.[1] Advanced structural and functional neuroimaging techniques have shed new light on these alterations. Although techniques such as PET and magnetoencephalography have also been used in an attempt to understand these changes, this article reviews functional MR imaging (fMR imaging) and diffusion tensor imaging (DTI) techniques. A brief discussion

of the use of advanced MR imaging techniques in the diagnosis of Meniere disease (MD) and dural arteriovenous fistulae (DAVF) is also presented.

NEURAL CORRELATES OF TINNITUS

Although tinnitus may originate from damage to peripheral auditory structures, it is well established that the perception of the phantom sound is largely the result of central neural processes. Evidence for a central origin of tinnitus stems from the finding that tinnitus is an invariable consequence of sectioning the auditory nerve, as may occur with acoustic neuroma surgery, and in such patients, tinnitus does not resolve and may actually worsen after the procedure.[1,2] Damage to hair cells of the inner ear related to age and noise exposure is the inciting process in most patients. Tinnitus is

Disclosure Statement: The authors have nothing to disclose.
Conflicts of Interest: None.
[a] Division of Neuroradiology, Department of Diagnostic Radiology and Nuclear Medicine, University of Maryland School of Medicine, 22 South Greene Street, Baltimore, MD 21201, USA; [b] Department of Radiology, University of Pittsburgh School of Medicine, Pittsburgh, PA, USA; [c] Division of Interventional Neuroradiology, University of Maryland School of Medicine, 22 South Greene Street, Baltimore, MD 21201, USA; [d] Departments of Radiology, Neurology and Neurosurgery, University of Maryland School of Medicine, 22 South Greene Street, Baltimore, MD 21201, USA
* Corresponding author.
E-mail address: praghavan@umm.edu

neuroimaging.theclinics.com

believed to arise from an abnormal neuroplastic response to this process, which manifests as hyperactivity of neurons at multiple levels in the auditory pathway. This hyperactivity may be the result either of central downregulation of inhibition,[3] or possibly from upregulation of excitatory inputs.[4] Reorganization of the auditory cortical tonotopic map[1] also is believed to occur. This results from cortical neurons deprived of auditory thalamocortical input responding to input from their unaffected neighbors.[5] The mechanisms responsible for how the phantom sound is consciously perceived remain elusive. Llinás and colleagues[6] propose that aberrant thalamocortical rhythms (thalamocortical dysrhythmia) that may emerge as a plastic maladaptation to peripheral auditory injury may generate the conscious percept of tinnitus. Changes in the brain with tinnitus are not confined to the auditory pathway. Roberts and colleagues[1] discuss the role of the somatosensory system in the modulation of the tinnitus percept, given that patients with tinnitus can alter their perception of the phantom sound by somatic maneuvers such as jaw clenching[7] or tensing their neck muscles. It is not surprising that changes in the limbic system are a feature of chronic tinnitus.[8–10] The hippocampus, nucleus accumbens, and amygdala, among others, seem to play a key role in the symptoms of anxiety, sleeplessness, and impairment of mood and memory that chronic tinnitus sufferers experience. For detailed discussion on the neural underpinnings of tinnitus, (See Ryan D, Bauer CA: Neuroscience of tinnitus, in this issue.)

FUNCTIONAL MR IMAGING IN TINNITUS

Since the discovery of the functional significance of spontaneous low-frequency blood oxygen level–dependent (BOLD) signal fluctuations (less than 0.1 Hz) in the brain by Biswal and colleagues,[11] the use of resting-state fMR imaging (rsfMR imaging) in neurologic disorders has greatly expanded. In this study, using a seed-based approach, a high degree of correlation in the temporal course of fluctuations between the left somatosensory cortex at rest and homologous areas in the right hemisphere was observed, comprising a functionally connected sensorimotor network. The physiologic basis for these temporal fluctuations is not entirely clear but seems to be tightly coupled with neural activity.[12] Several other resting-state networks (RSNs) have been subsequently discovered. Of these, the default mode network (DMN) discovered by Raichle and colleagues[13] on PET imaging, and then by Greicius and colleagues[14] on rsfMR imaging, is perhaps the best known. In addition, RSNs for language, memory, vision, hearing, and attention, among others, have been identified and examined in depth.

Several methods may be used to extract networks from resting-state data. After undergoing a series of preprocessing steps, including correction for section-dependent time shifts and intensity differences, head motion, nuisance regression (related to cardiac and respiratory motion), spatial smoothing, application of low-pass filters, and registration to standardized atlas space, data may be analyzed using a seed-based approach, independent component analysis (ICA), or graph methods among other techniques.[15] Each of these has its strengths and weaknesses. The seed-based approach, in which a region of interest (ROI) is placed over the area in question and its BOLD time series correlated with all other voxels in the brain, is perhaps the most frequently used method. However, this approach requires a priori selection of ROIs. ICA is also a widely used method that is perhaps statistically more robust, requiring fewer a priori assumptions. These approaches are comparable. Rosazza and colleagues[16] in a resting-state study of 40 participants found significant (though not complete) correspondence between these methods. Graph theory methods allow representation of ROIs as a network of nodes and edges from which several connectional characteristics may be inferred. Graph methods have revealed that the brain's intrinsic activity is organized as a small-world, highly efficient network, with significant modularity and highly connected hub regions.[15,17]

fMR imaging studies in tinnitus reveal 2 broad themes: correlation differences between auditory and nonauditory brain networks, and an increased correlation between the limbic system and other brain areas. These, discussed in detail in an excellent review of the topic by Husain and Schmidt,[18] reflect to a large extent what is now understood about the neural correlates of tinnitus. Aberrant neural activity in auditory and nonauditory regions has been described in numerous studies.[19,20] In a task-based fMR imaging study, Golm and colleagues[21] describe increased activity in a fronto-parietal-cingulate network, which seems to be more active in highly distressed tinnitus patients. In a group of 13 patients with chronic tinnitus, Maudoux and colleagues[20] describe increased connectivity in extra-auditory regions such as the brainstem, cerebellum, nucleus accumbens, parahippocampal gyrus, and sensorimotor cortex, indicating a modification of cortical and subcortical functional connectivity to include areas that participate in attention, memory, and emotional processes.

Support for alterations in memory networks may also be found in single-photon emission computed tomography (SPECT) studies. For example, Laureano and colleagues[22] describe significantly increased perfusion in the parahippocampal gyrus using SPECT, in a series of 20 subjects with chronic tinnitus and normal hearing. Interactions between the auditory and limbic systems using fMR imaging have been revealed in studies by Kim and Horwitz,[23] and discussed in a review by Rauschecker and colleagues.[24] The role of visual and attentional networks has been explored by Burton and colleagues.[25] In a study of 17 subjects with bothersome tinnitus, negative correlations reciprocally characterized functional connectivity between auditory and occipital-visual cortex. Connectivity for primary visual cortex in tinnitus included extensive negative correlations with regions that participate in the executive control network. The investigators interpret this dissociation in activity between the auditory cortex and visual and attention-control networks in 2 ways: either the reciprocal negative correlations in connectivity between these networks are a maladaptation or they reflect an adaptive response to suppress the salience of the phantom sound and minimize conflict with attentional tasks. In an rsfMR imaging study by Schmidt and colleagues,[26] in subjects with tinnitus and mild-to-moderate high-frequency hearing loss, the DMN was the only RSN to display visual differences between subjects with tinnitus and controls. In the DMN, strongly decreased correlation was identified between seed regions and the precuneus. Using a seed-based approach, in the same study, increased connectivity was noted between limbic areas (the left parahippocampal gyrus) and the auditory RSN and the attention network (right parahippocampal gyrus).

The investigators suggest that treatment strategies aimed at relieving tinnitus-related distress target increased limbic-auditory or attention network connectivity, as well as the decreased coherence of the DMN. Disruption of the DMN may be attributable to changes in the middle temporal and angular gyri, as evidenced by increased amplitude of low-frequency fluctuation (ALFF),[27] a measure that may reflect the intensity of regional spontaneous brain activity found in these areas by Chen and colleagues.[19] They also found increased ALFF in the superior frontal gyrus, a finding that correlated with the duration of tinnitus. This may lend support to the hypothesis that the frontal cortex may be a vital structure subserving the tinnitus mechanism, as proposed by Jastreboff.[28] Chen and colleagues[19] also found decreased ALFF values in the visual cortex and

thalami. The decreased visual cortical ALFF may be a consequence of suppression of the visual network by the phantom sounds, whereas the thalamic alterations may be a manifestation of the thalamocortical dysrhythmia hypothesis of Llinás and colleagues.[6] Fig. 1 provides a summary of recent fMR imaging studies in tinnitus.

It must be stressed that the findings of fMR imaging studies must be interpreted with a measure of caution. Variations in the analytical methods used (eg, seed-based methods vs ICA) in the anatomic locations of ROIs studied and in the numbers of subjects evaluated may all affect results. Husain and colleagues[18] recommend that researchers focused on the use of rsfMR imaging in tinnitus voluntarily adopt a more standardized approach in the design of their fMR imaging studies. The effect of mechanical noise intrinsic to MR imaging scanners, despite the use of noise reduction strategies, also cannot be disregarded.[18] However, the most important variable may be the heterogeneity in the clinical characteristics of subjects studied.[18] These may lie in demographic features (eg, age, gender) or in the

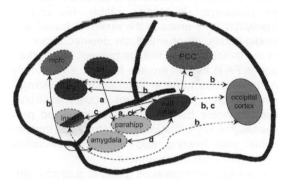

Fig. 1. Main results of resting-state functional connectivity studies in tinnitus. The major networks highlighted are default-mode (*blue*), limbic (*green*), auditory (*red*), the visual (*orange*), and several attention networks (specifically dorsal attention and the executive control of attention; *purple*). Positive correlations between regions that are stronger in tinnitus subjects than controls are shown in solid lines and negative correlations are dashed lines. Modifications to the networks do not represent the networks in their entirety. Connections are labeled representing the studies in which they were reported: (a) Schmidt and colleagues,[26] (b) Burton and colleagues,[25] (c) Maudoux and colleagues,[2] and (d) Kim and colleagues.[23] Aud cortex, auditory cortex; fef, frontal eye fields; lifg, left inferior frontal gyrus; mpfc, medial prefrontal cortex; parahipp, parahippocampus; PCC, posterior cingulate cortex. (*From* Husain FT, Schmidt SA. Using resting-state functional connectivity to unravel networks of tinnitus. Hear Res 2014:307;153–62; with permission.)

clinical characteristics of the tinnitus itself (eg, severity, laterality, associated hearing loss). The importance of recognizing this variability was also recognized by Wineland and colleagues.[29] In a study of 18 subjects with nonbothersome tinnitus, they found no alterations in functional connectivity of the auditory cortex or of other relevant cortical areas. This was in contrast to an earlier study by Burton and colleagues[25] in which changes in connectivity of sensory and cognitive networks were observed in a cohort of subjects with bothersome tinnitus. The investigators stress that imaging studies that recognize the heterogeneity of the cognitive and emotional symptoms that accompany tinnitus may be more informative than those that do not.

ADVANCED STRUCTURAL IMAGING

In one of the earliest studies exploring the role of DTI in tinnitus, Lee and colleagues[30] described a small, yet statistically significant decrease in fractional anisotropy (FA) values in the left frontal and right parietal arcuate fasciculi in a group of 28 patients. They postulated that the percept of tinnitus may be related to alterations in specific white matter pathways. Of these, notably, the arcuate fasciculus links areas in the auditory, frontal and limbic cortex, all of which are deemed important in the genesis of the tinnitus percept. The reduction in FA in the left arcuate fasciculus may imply a "lack of harmony in information processing," whereas changes in the right arcuate fasciculus may implicate the role of attention-related processes.[30] A key limitation of this study was that patients with hearing loss were not evaluated separately from those without.

In a more homogeneous group of subjects, Aldhafeeri and colleagues[31] found significant correlations between cortical thickness reductions in the bilateral temporal and frontal lobes of subjects with tinnitus. This reduction was present to a greater degree in subjects with associated hearing loss. These differences were most evident in the prefrontal cortex, temporal lobes, and limbic system. The investigators postulate that the decreased prefrontal cortical thickness, in conjunction with the decreased FA that was found in the inferior fronto-occipital fasciculus, may be central to the deficits in cognition, attention, emotional, and memory deficits experienced by tinnitus sufferers. The investigators also noted decreased FA in the inferior longitudinal fasciculus (which may mediate visual-limbic interactions) and in the corpus callosal splenium, perhaps manifesting as an imbalance between interhemispheric excitation and inhibition. They also describe a

reduction in cortical thickness in the auditory cortex, supporting studies by Schneider and colleagues,[32] who used voxel-based morphometry to demonstrate decreased gray matter thickness in Heschl gyrus.[26]

In a DTI study, Crippa and colleagues[33] found increased connectivity between the amygdala and the auditory cortex, implying increased auditory-limbic interaction in tinnitus sufferers. In this small study of 10 subjects, associated hearing deficits were not accounted for. In a 2011 study, Husain and colleagues[34] found that hearing loss, rather than tinnitus itself, may have a more significant impact on gray and white matter changes as detected by voxel-based morphometry and DTI. Studies that effectively combine structural and functional neuroimaging methods to evaluate the neural basis of tinnitus are scarce. In their review, Husain and colleagues[18] stress the need for such work, ideally conducted on a clinically homogeneous population.

MENIERE DISEASE

MD is characterized by intermittent episodes of vertigo (with horizontal rotatory nystagmus), fluctuating sensorineural hearing loss, tinnitus, and aural pressure.[35] Intense tinnitus is common in MD and is more often seen in the late stage of the disease.[36,37] The causes of MD and the pathologic changes in the inner ear during acute exacerbations of MD are incompletely understood. Dilatation of the endolymphatic spaces (hydrops) of the inner ear arising from obstruction to endolymph outflow in the endolymphatic sac and duct is a basic pathologic feature of MD. The histologic processes that affect the sac or duct include perisaccular fibrosis, loss of saccular epithelial integrity, and atrophy or hypoplasia of the vestibular duct.[35] There also seems to be an association between a more anteromedially placed sigmoid sinus and development of MD, perhaps as a result of vascular compression of the endolymphatic sac.[38] A diagnosis of MD may be challenging, given the intermittent nature of its symptomatology. MD may be typical when the full spectrum of cochlear (hearing loss with tinnitus and a sensation of aural pressure) and vestibular (vertigo with aural pressure) symptoms are present and atypical when only 1 or the other is experienced. MD is usually diagnosed by clinical means (Box 1) with a certain diagnosis being possible only when histopathological evidence of endolymphatic hydrops (ELH) is available.

MR imaging is obtained when a diagnosis of MD is equivocal, with the intent of excluding other retrocochlear disease. Of late, MR imaging techniques capable of demonstrating ELH in the minute compartments of the inner ear have emerged. The inner ear contains 2 types of fluid: perilymph (with an ionic composition similar to cerebrospinal fluid and plasma, contained within the scala vestibuli and scala tympani of the cochlea) and endolymph (with a higher potassium ion concentration than perilymph, contained within the membranous labyrinth), separated by a watertight membrane to preserve electrolyte hemostasis.[39] The ability to differentiate endolymph from perilymph using MR imaging enhanced with gadolinium diethylenetriamine pentaacetic acid–bismethylamide (Gd-DTPA-BMA) was reported by Counter and colleagues[40] and the mechanisms of Gd-DTPA-BMA transport in the inner ear were elucidated by Zou and colleagues.[41] Gadolinium-based contrast media may be administered intravenously or intratympanically. In guinea pig

models of MD, both modes of administration resulted in accumulation of contrast in the perilymphatic spaces but not in the endolymph. In animal models with ELH, bulging of the Reissner membrane was observed as a deficit of contrast medium in the scala vestibuli.[42]

Although gadolinium-based contrast media may be delivered to the inner ear via intravenous and intratympanic injection, from a clinical standpoint, intravenous administration is perhaps more practical and may result in contrast accumulation in the inner ear in a more homogeneous and rapid fashion. The homogeneity of contrast distribution may be especially important given recent concerns of altered intratympanic contrast agent distribution via the round window in patients with MD. The intratympanic method may be safer due to limited systemic dispersion, especially in patients with impaired renal function.[43,44] ELH in patients with MD, evident as expansion of the endolymphatic spaces devoid of contrast medium after intratympanic administration has been demonstrated in several studies. In a recent study, Barath and colleagues[45] were able to identify ELH in 73% of ears of patients with possible MD, in 100% of ears with probable MD, and 95% of ears with definite MD, with a 3-dimensional (3D) real inversion recovery sequence obtained 4 hours after intravenous contrast administration. They also developed a simple clinically relevant grading system for hydrops with a high degree of interobserver agreement. Homann and colleagues[43] observed a correlation between symptom severity and the degree of ELH 4 hours after intravenous application of a single dose of gadobutrol (Gd-DO3A-butrol), using highly T2-weighted fluid attenuation inversion recovery (FLAIR) and T2 driven equilibrium sequences. These sequences permit derivation of positive perilymphatic images (PPIs) and positive endolymphatic images (PEIs). Subtraction of PEI from PPI, using techniques described by Naganawa and colleagues,[46] yields hybrid of reversed image of positive endolymph signal and native image of positive perilymph signal (HYDROPS) images (Fig. 2). These images were then evaluated for ELH using semiquantitative and volumetric methods, with the former proving to be highly accurate.

ADVANCED IMAGING OF DURAL ARTERIOVENOUS FISTULAE

Dural AVFs reportedly account for up to 20% of all cases of pulse synchronous tinnitus.[47,48] Catheter angiography remains the gold standard for the diagnosis of DAVF but is not without risk.[49] It is important, therefore, when evaluating

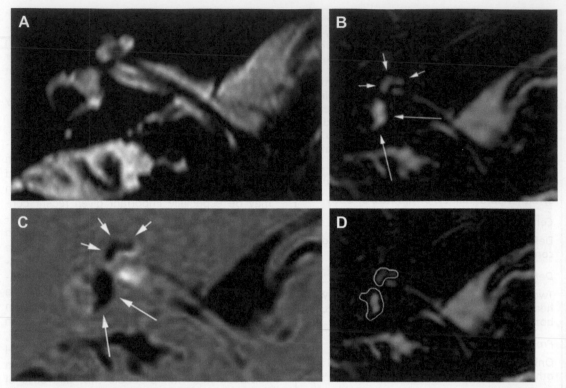

Fig. 2. A 57-year-old woman with Meniere disease, 4 hours after intravenous administration of a single dose of Gd-DO3A-butrol. (*A*) T2DRIVE-cisternography reveals the anatomy of the total lymphatic fluid of the right inner ear. (*B*) Heavily T2-weighted FLAIR PEI with an inversion time of 2050 ms displays the endolymphatic fluid. (*C*) The HYDROPS image, gained by subtraction of PEI from PPI, reveals the enlarged endolymphatic space as black area. Diagnosis after semiquantitative analysis was a significant (II°) ELH of the vestibule (*long arrows*) and the cochlea (*short arrows*). Volumetric assessment was performed by dedicated slice-by-slice-segmentation of the endolymphatic space in PEI (*D*) and the total labyrinth fluid space in T2DRIVE-cisternography. This patient showed an endolymph or total labyrinthine fluid-ratio of 50.51% (cochlea) and 54.3% (vestibule). (*From* Homann G, Vieth V, Weiss D, et al. Semi-quantitative vs volumetric determination of endolymphatic space in Meniere's disease using endolymphatic hydrops 3T-HR-MRI after intravenous gadolinium injection. PLoS One 2015;10(3):e0120357.")

cross-sectional imaging studies of patients with pulse synchronous tinnitus, to be aware of signs that may indicate the presence of a DAVF. In a short case series of 7 subjects with pulsatile tinnitus, Narvid and colleagues[50] described several direct and indirect signs on computed tomography angiography (CTA) that may suggest a diagnosis of intracranial DAVF. The presence of abnormally enlarged arterial feeding vessels was reported to be a specific and sensitive marker for this entity. However, other findings, such as asymmetrically increased draining veins, the presence of transcalvarial channels, a shaggy appearance of the tentorium and adjacent venous sinuses, and the presence of prominent cortical venous channels, were not sensitive enough. Refinements in CTA technology, such as the use of 320-section scanners that permit performance of dynamic 4-dimensional (4D)-CTA may permit identification and classification of DAVFs,

comparable to what may be achieved with catheter angiography.[51,52] Full agreement between 4D-CTA and digital subtraction angiography (DSA) was demonstrated in 10 out of 11 subjects by Willems and colleagues,[53] who cautioned that small slow-flow fistulae may not be demonstrable by the former technique. In a series of 29 subjects with DAVF, 4D-CTA was able to identify 32 out of 33 DSA-confirmed fistula and was also able to accurately grade 31 out of 33 by the Cognard classification.[54]

Tracking of a bolus of contrast medium through the cerebral vasculature is also possible with time-resolved MR angiography (trMRA) techniques (**Fig. 3**).[55] Meckel and colleagues[56] reported that 3D-trMRA correctly detected the side and presence of all patent fistulae in a series of 14 subjects. The reliability of trMRA as a screening and surveillance tool in a larger series of 40 subjects was also described by Farb and colleagues,[57] who

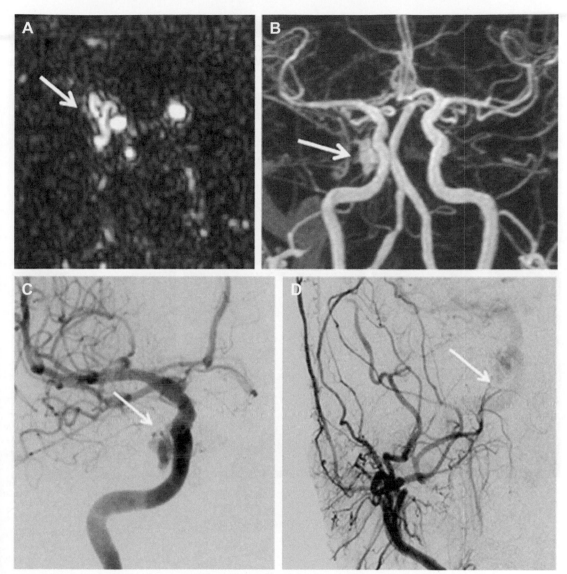

Fig. 3. trMRA of an indirect right carotid cavernous fistula in a patient with pulse synchronous tinnitus. (*A*) Axial image obtained using a time-resolved imaging of contrast kinetics (TRICKS) sequence demonstrating enhancement in the right cavernous sinus (*arrow*) due to AV shunting, implying the presence of a fistula. (*B*) A maximum intensity projection reconstruction demonstrating enhancement in the right cavernous sinus (*arrow*). The internal (*C*) and external (*D*) carotid catheter angiograms confirm the presence of a type D indirect carotid-cavernous fistula (*arrows*) supplied by the inferolateral and meningohypophyseal trunks and by meningeal branches of the internal maxillary artery.

demonstrated that in 93% of their cases, trMRA facilitated correct identification (or exclusion) and classification of fistulae. More recently, using a time-resolved imaging of contrast kinetics (TRICKS) sequence on a 1.5 T MR imaging scanner, Pekkola and Kangasniemi[58] described sensitivity and specificity of 94.4% and 83.3%, respectively, for detection of early arterial filling in a series of 19 subjects with posterior fossa fistulae. Good-to-excellent agreement with DSA was described using a 4D contrast-enhanced MR

angiography (MRA) technique on a 3T scanner by Nishimura and colleagues.[59] They attributed such agreement to the relatively high spatial and temporal resolution of their technique, which used parallel imaging with keyhole acquisition and a segmented contrast-enhanced timing-robust angiography (CENTRA), a central k-space ordering, k-space sampling, technique.

Susceptibility-weighted imaging (SWI) has also been applied to the diagnosis of DAVF. In a short report, Letourneau-Guillon and colleagues[60] were able identify the site of fistulization in 5 out of 6 subjects, depicted as hyperintense venous signal, but were limited in their ability to identify cortical venous reflux. However, venous congestion, seen as a pseudophlebitic pattern on DSA, correlated anatomically with increased number, caliber, and tortuosity of hypointense veins seen on SWI. SWI was found to be superior to conventional

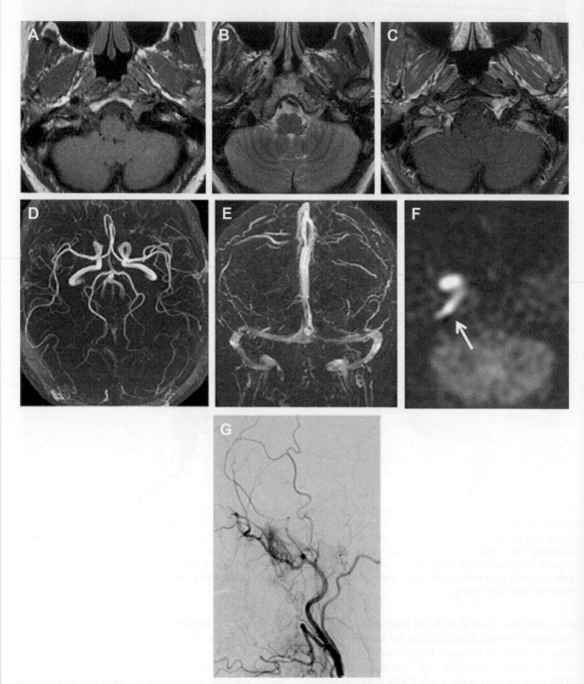

Fig. 4. Right infratemporal fossa arteriovenous malformation (AVM) on ASL in a 56-year-old patient with recent onset of pulse synchronous tinnitus. Note the lack of abnormality on the conventional T1 (*A*), T2 (*B*), and post-contrast T1-weighted (*C*) images. The MRA and MR venography (*D* and *E*) were also unrevealing. The axial ASL image (*F*), however, demonstrates high signal intensity–labeled spins in the pterygoid veins inferior to the skull base (*arrow*), indicating the presence of arteriovenous shunting. The external carotid artery injection on a catheter angiogram (*G*) confirms the presence of an AVM, supplied by the internal maxillary artery. (*Courtesy* of NJ Fischbein, MD, Palo Alto, CA.)

MR imaging in the detection of venous congestion. Therefore, they suggested an important role for SWI in the detection and assessment of the hemodynamics associated with DAVFs.[60] Noguchi and colleagues[61] were also able to demonstrate dilated cerebral veins in all of their 14 DAVF subjects, which corresponded well with areas of increased cerebral blood volume on dynamic susceptibility contrast imaging.

Arterial spin-labeling (ASL) is an MR imaging perfusion method that has recently been used for the detection of DAVFs.[62] ASL, a noninvasive technique that does not require administration of gadolinium-based contrast, can provide

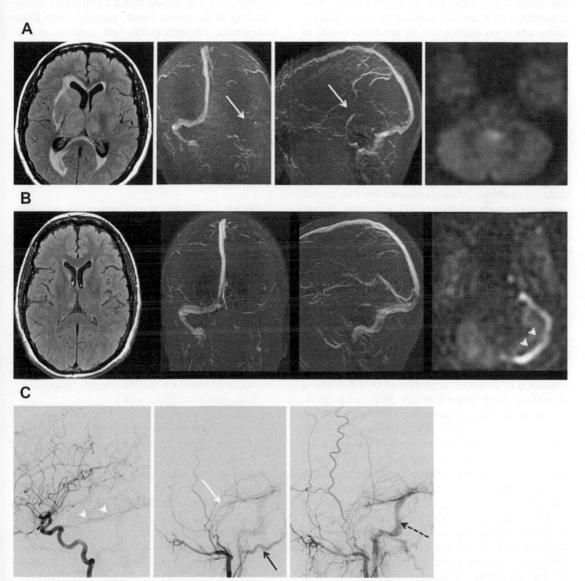

Fig. 5. Value of ASL in pulse synchronous tinnitus. (A) Axial FLAIR, MRV, MRA, and ASL images, from left to right, respectively, in a 42-year-old woman who presented acutely with confusion and lethargy. These demonstrate thalamic and basal ganglia edema due to thrombosis of the deep cerebral venous system and of the left transverse sinus. Note the lack of any abnormally increased signal in the ASL image. (B) Axial FLAIR, MRV, MRA, and ASL images, from left to right, respectively, obtained 6 months after resolution of the acute episode, when the patient presented with new pulsatile tinnitus. The basal ganglia and thalamic edema has resolved and the deep venous system has recanalized. Note however, the appearance of high venous signal in the left transverse sinus in the ASL image (arrowheads). The catheter angiogram (C) demonstrates an AV fistula supplied by branches of the meningohypophyseal trunk (arrowheads), parietal branches of the middle meningeal artery (white arrow) and the occipital artery (black arrow) with shunting into the transverse and sigmoid sinuses (dashed arrow). (Courtesy of NJ Fischbein, MD, Palo Alto, CA.)

quantitative assessment of cerebral blood flow (expressed in units of ml/100 g/min) by using arterial water as a freely diffusible tracer.[63] An inversion pulse is applied to tag inflowing blood water spins proximal to the volume of interest. Following a transit delay to permit tagged spins to circulate within the imaging plane and exchange with tissue, control and label images are obtained. After acquisition of a certain number of such images, these are then subtracted to produce maps of brain perfusion.[63] Although arterial spins may be labeled using continuous, pulsed, and velocity-selective methods, a modification of the continuous method (pseudocontinuous ASL [PCASL], which provides superior labeling efficiency and is compatible with modern coil hardware) is recommended for clinical imaging.[64] ASL was applied by Wolf and colleagues[65] to demonstrate arteriovenous shunting in cerebral vascular malformations. The T1 relaxation of labeled arterial water is relatively short compared with its transit time, and most labeled blood will relax during transit through capillaries, before exchange with brain tissue water. In normal circumstances, therefore, after its passage through the capillary bed, there is minimal venous outflow of label; however, in arteriovenous malformations due to the presence of a shunt (absence of a normal capillary bed), this leads to the nidus and draining veins demonstrating increased contrast[65] (Fig. 4). Extending this principle to DAVFs, Le and colleagues[62] demonstrated increased signal in draining veins (Fig. 5) as a strong predictor of the presence of a fistula as confirmed by DSA with a sensitivity and specificity of 78% and 85%, respectively. They recommend including ASL as a part of a routine MR imaging protocol for intracerebral hemorrhage and in circumstances such as patients with pulsatile tinnitus for whom a small arteriovenous malformation or fistula is a concern.

Despite these exciting advances, catheter angiography retains its status as the definitive modality in the evaluation of DAVF, given its excellent spatial and temporal resolution, its ability to delineate all aspects of the complex hemodynamic features of this entity, and the guidance it provides in the planning of endovascular or surgical treatment.[55]

SUMMARY

As Wineland and colleagues[29] show, tinnitus is more than just ringing in the ear and is associated with a host of distressing nonauditory symptoms. The neural networks responsible for its genesis, perception, and attendant symptomatology are incompletely understood but are beginning to be unraveled using several advanced noninvasive imaging techniques. Although a growing body of literature has begun to accumulate on this topic, results must be interpreted recognizing the heterogeneity of this disorder. Also, a need for standardizing study protocols exists. Tinnitus remains an intractable problem and it is hoped that an improved understanding of its neural basis, derived from these techniques, will help guide new, promising neuromodulatory therapies targeting specific brain regions.

ACKNOWLEDGMENTS

We would like to thank Brigitte Pocta MLA for her assistance with formatting of this article.

REFERENCES

1. Roberts LE, Eggermont JJ, Caspary DM, et al. Ringing ears: the neuroscience of tinnitus. J Neurosci 2010;30(45):14972–9.
2. House JW, Brackmann DE. Tinnitus: surgical treatment. Ciba Found Symp 1981;85:204–16.
3. Middleton JW, Tzounopoulos T. Imaging the neural correlates of tinnitus: a comparison between animal models and human studies. Front Syst Neurosci 2012;6:35.
4. Dehmel S, Pradhan S, Koehler S, et al. Noise overexposure alters long-term somatosensory-auditory processing in the dorsal cochlear nucleus—possible basis for tinnitus-related hyperactivity? J Neurosci 2012;32(5):1660–71.
5. Eggermont JJ, Roberts LE. The neuroscience of tinnitus. Trends Neurosci 2004;27(11):676–82.
6. Llinás R, Urbano FJ, Leznik E, et al. Rhythmic and dysrhythmic thalamocortical dynamics: GABA systems and the edge effect. Trends Neurosci 2005; 28(6):325–33.
7. Pinchoff RJ, Burkard RF, Salvi RJ, et al. Modulation of tinnitus by voluntary jaw movements. Am J Otol 1998;19(6):785–9.
8. De Ridder D, Fransen H, Francois O, et al. Amygdalohippocampal involvement in tinnitus and auditory memory. Acta Otolaryngol Suppl 2006;566:50–3.
9. Landgrebe M, Langguth B, Rosengarth B, et al. Structural brain changes in tinnitus: grey matter decrease in auditory and non-auditory brain areas. Neuroimage 2009;46:213–8.
10. Lockwood AH, Salvi RJ, Coad ML, et al. The functional neuroanatomy of tinnitus: evidence for limbic system links and neural plasticity. Neurology 1998; 50:114–20.
11. Biswal B, Yetkin FZ, Haughton VM, et al. Functional connectivity in the motor cortex of resting human

brain using echo-planar MRI. Magnetic resonance in medicine 1995;34(4):537–41.

12. Schölvinck ML, Maier A, Ye FQ, et al. Neural basis of global resting-state fMRI activity. Proc Natl Acad Sci U S A 2010;107(22):10238–43.

13. Raichle M, MacLeod A, Snyder A, et al. A default mode of brain function. Proc Natl Acad Sci U S A 2001;98:676–82.

14. Greicius M, Krasnow B, Reiss A, et al. Functional connectivity in the resting brain: a network analysis of the default mode hypothesis. Proc Natl Acad Sci U S A 2003;100:253–8.

15. Lee MH, Smyser CD, Shimony JS. Resting-state fMRI: a review of methods and clinical applications. AJNR Am J Neuroradiol 2013;34(10):1866–72.

16. Rosazza C, Minati L, Ghielmetti F, et al. Functional connectivity during resting-state functional MR imaging: study of the correspondence between independent component analysis and region-of-interest-based methods. AJNR Am J Neuroradiol 2012;33:180–7.

17. Wang J, Zuo X, He Y. Graph-based network analysis of resting-state functional MRI. Front Syst Neurosci 2010;4:16.

18. Husain FT, Schmidt SA. Using resting state functional connectivity to unravel networks of tinnitus. Hear Res 2014;307:153–62.

19. Chen YC, Zhang J, Li XW, et al. Aberrant spontaneous brain activity in chronic tinnitus patients revealed by resting-state functional MRI. Neuroimage Clin 2014;6:222–8.

20. Maudoux A, Lefebvre P, Cabay JE, et al. Connectivity graph analysis of the auditory resting state network in tinnitus. Brain Res 2012;1485:10–21.

21. Golm D, Schmidt-Samoa C, Dechent P, et al. Neural correlates of tinnitus related distress: an fMRI-study. Hear Res 2013;295:87–99.

22. Laureano MR, Onishi ET, Bressan RA, et al. Memory networks in tinnitus: a functional brain image study. PLoS One 2014;9(2):e87839.

23. Kim J, Horwitz B. How well does structural equation modeling reveal abnormal brain anatomical connections? an fMRI simulation study. Neuroimage 2009;45:1190–8.

24. Rauschecker JP, Leaver AM, Muhlau M. Tuning out the noise: limbic-auditory interactions in tinnitus. Neuron 2010;66:819–26.

25. Burton H, Wineland A, Bhattacharya M, et al. Altered networks in bothersome tinnitus: a functional connectivity study. BMC Neurosci 2012;13(1):3.

26. Schmidt SA, Akrofi K, Carpenter-Thompson JR, et al. Default mode, dorsal attention and auditory resting state networks exhibit differential functional connectivity in tinnitus and hearing loss. PLoS One 2013;8(10):e76488.

27. Zou QH, Zhu CZ, Yang Y, et al. An improved approach to detection of amplitude of low-frequency fluctuation (ALFF) for resting-state fMRI: fractional ALFF. J Neurosci Methods 2008;172(1):137–41.

28. Jastreboff PJ. Phantom auditory perception (tinnitus): mechanisms of generation and perception. Neurosci Res 1990;8(4):221–54.

29. Wineland AM, Burton H, Piccirillo J. Functional connectivity networks in nonbothersome tinnitus. Otolaryngol Head Neck Surg 2012;145(5):900–6.

30. Lee YJ, Bae SJ, Lee SH, et al. Evaluation of white matter structures in patients with tinnitus using diffusion tensor imaging. J Clin Neurosci 2007;14(6):515–9.

31. Aldhafeeri FM, Mackenzie I, Kay T, et al. Neuroanatomical correlates of tinnitus revealed by cortical thickness analysis and diffusion tensor imaging. Neuroradiology 2012;54(8):883–92.

32. Schneider P, Andermann M, Wengenroth M, et al. Reduced volume of Heschl's gyrus in tinnitus. Neuroimage 2009;45(3):927–39.

33. Crippa A, Lanting CP, Van Dijk P, et al. A diffusion tensor imaging study on the auditory system and tinnitus. Open Neuroimag J 2010;4:16–25.

34. Husain FT, Medina RE, Davis CW, et al. Neuroanatomical changes due to hearing loss and chronic tinnitus: a combined VBM and DTI study. Brain Res 2011;1369:74–88.

35. Sajjadi H, Paparella MM. Meniere's disease. Lancet 2008;372(9636):406–14.

36. Committee on Hearing and Equilibrium guidelines for the diagnosis and evaluation of therapy in Meniere's disease otolaryngology American Academy of Otolaryngology-Head and Neck Foundation, Inc. Otolaryngol Head Neck Surg 1995;113:181–5.

37. Havia M, Kentala E, Pyykkö I. Hearing loss and tinnitus in Meniere's disease. Auris Nasus Larynx 2002;29(2):115–9.

38. Paparella MM, Sajjadi H, da Costa SS, et al. The significance of the lateral sinus in Meniere's disease. In: Nadol JB, editor. Proc 2nd Intl Symposium on Meniere's Disease: Pathogenesis, Pathophysiology, Diagnosis, and Treatment. Amsterdam: Kugler Publications; 1989. p. 139–46.

39. Leonova EV, Raphael Y. Organization of cell junctions and cytoskeleton in the reticular lamina in normal and ototoxically damaged organ of Corti. Hear Res 1997;113:14–28.

40. Counter SA, Bjelke B, Klason T, et al. Magnetic resonance imaging of the cochlea, spiral ganglia and eighth nerve of the guinea pig. Neuroreport 1999;10:473–9.

41. Zou J, Pyykkö I, Counter SA, et al. In vivo observation of dynamic perilymph formation using 4.7 T MRI with gadolinium as a tracer. Acta Otolaryngol 2003;123:910–5.

42. Pyykkö I, Zou J, Poe D, et al. Magnetic resonance imaging of the inner ear in Meniere's disease. Otolaryngol Clin North Am 2010;43(5):1059–80.

43. Homann G, Vieth V, Weiss D, et al. Semi-quantitative vs. volumetric determination of endolymphatic space in Menière's disease using endolymphatic hydrops 3T-HR-MRI after intravenous gadolinium injection. PLoS One 2015;10(3):e0120357.

44. Shi H, Li Y, Yin S, et al. The predominant vestibular uptake of gadolinium through the oval window pathway is compromised by endolymphatic hydrops in Meniere's disease. Otol Neurotol 2014;35:315–22.

45. Barath K, Schuknecht B, Naldi AM, et al. Detection and grading of endolymphatic hydrops in Meniere disease using MR imaging. AJNR Am J Neuroradiol 2014;35(7):1387–92.

46. Naganawa S, Yamazaki M, Kawai H, et al. Imaging of Meniere's disease after intravenous administration of single-dose gadodiamide: utility of subtraction images with different inversion time. Magn Reson Med Sci 2012;11:213–9.

47. Waldvogel D, Mattle HP, Sturzenegger M, et al. Pulsatile tinnitus–a review of 84 patients. J Neurol 1998; 245(3):137–42.

48. Sonmez G, Basekim CC, Ozturk E, et al. Imaging of pulsatile tinnitus: a review of 74 patients. Clin Imaging 2007;31:102–8.

49. Kaufmann TJ, Huston J III, Mandrekar JN, et al. Complications of diagnostic cerebral angiography: evaluation of 19,826 consecutive patients. Radiology 2007;243(3):812–9.

50. Narvid J, Do HM, Blevins NH, et al. CT angiography as a screening tool for dural arteriovenous fistula in patients with pulsatile tinnitus: feasibility and test characteristics. AJNR Am J Neuroradiol 2011;32(3):446–53.

51. Brouwer PA, Bosman T, Van Walderveen MAA, et al. Dynamic 320-section CT angiography in cranial arteriovenous shunting lesions. AJNR Am J Neuroradiol 2010;31(4):767–70.

52. Kortman HGJ, Smit EJ, Oei MTH, et al. 4D-CTA in neurovascular disease: a review. AJNR Am J Neuroradiol 2015;36(6):1026–33.

53. Willems PWA, Brouwer PA, Barfett JJ, et al. Detection and classification of cranial dural arteriovenous fistulas using 4D-CT angiography: initial experience. AJNR Am J Neuroradiol 2011;32(1):49–53.

54. Fujiwara H, Momoshima S, Akiyama T, et al. Whole-brain CT digital subtraction angiography of cerebral dural arteriovenous fistula using 320-detector row CT. Neuroradiology 2013;55(7):837–43.

55. Miller TR, Gandhi D. Intracranial dural arteriovenous fistulae: clinical presentation and management strategies. Stroke 2015;46(7):2017–25.

56. Meckel S, Maier M, Ruiz DSM, et al. MR angiography of dural arteriovenous fistulas: diagnosis and follow-up after treatment using a time-resolved 3D contrast-enhanced technique. AJNR Am J Neuroradiol 2007;28(5):877–84.

57. Farb RI, Agid R, Willinsky RA, et al. Cranial dural arteriovenous fistula: diagnosis and classification with time-resolved MR angiography at 3T. AJNR Am J Neuroradiol 2009;30(8):1546–51.

58. Pekkola J, Kangasniemi M. Posterior fossa dural arteriovenous fistulas: diagnosis and follow-up with time-resolved imaging of contrast kinetics (TRICKS) at 1.5 T. Acta Radiol 2011;52(4):442–7.

59. Nishimura S, Hirai T, Sasao A, et al. Evaluation of dural arteriovenous fistulas with 4D contrast-enhanced MR angiography at 3T. AJNR Am J Neuroradiol 2010;31(1):80–5.

60. Letourneau-Guillon L, Krings T. Simultaneous arteriovenous shunting and venous congestion identification in dural arteriovenous fistulas using susceptibility-weighted imaging: initial experience. AJNR Am J Neuroradiol 2012;33(2):301–7.

61. Noguchi K, Kuwayama N, Kubo M, et al. Intracranial dural arteriovenous fistula with retrograde cortical venous drainage: use of susceptibility-weighted imaging in combination with dynamic susceptibility contrast imaging. AJNR Am J Neuroradiol 2010; 31(10):1903–10.

62. Le TT, Fischbein NJ, Andre JB, et al. Identification of venous signal on arterial spin labeling improves diagnosis of dural arteriovenous fistulas and small arteriovenous malformations. AJNR Am J Neuroradiol 2012;33(1):61–8.

63. Deibler AR, Pollock JM, Kraft RA, et al. Arterial spin-labeling in routine clinical practice, part 1: technique and artifacts. AJNR Am J Neuroradiol 2008;29(7):1228–34.

64. Alsop DC, Detre JA, Golay X, et al. Recommended implementation of arterial spin-labeled perfusion MRI for clinical applications: a consensus of the ISMRM perfusion study group and the European consortium for ASL in dementia. Magn Reson Med 2015;73(1):102–16.

65. Wolf RL, Wang J, Detre JA, et al. Arteriovenous shunt visualization in arteriovenous malformations with arterial spin-labeling MR imaging. AJNR Am J Neuroradiol 2008;29(4):681–7.

Index

Note: Page numbers of article titles are in **boldface** type.

Neuroimag Clin N Am 26 (2016) 313–316
http://dx.doi.org/10.1016/S1052-5149(16)30023-5
1052-5149/16/$ – see front matter © 2016 Elsevier Inc. All rights reserved.

neuroimaging.theclinics.com

Printed and bound by CPI Group (UK) Ltd, Croydon, CR0 4YY

03/10/2024

01040304-0004